Advances in Fixation Technology for the Foot and Ankle

Guest Editor

PATRICK R. BURNS, DPM, FACFAS

CLINICS IN PODIATRIC MEDICINE AND SURGERY

www.podiatric.theclinics.com

Consulting Editor

THOMAS ZGONIS, DPM, FACFAS

October 2011 • Volume 28 • Number 4

SAUNDERS an imprint of ELSEVIER, Inc.

W.B. SAUNDERS COMPANY
A Division of Elsevier Inc.

1600 John F. Kennedy Boulevard • Suite 1800 • Philadelphia, Pennsylvania 19103-2899

http://www.theclinics.com

CLINICS IN PODIATRIC MEDICINE AND SURGERY Volume 28, Number 4
October 2011 ISSN 0891-8422, ISBN-13: 978-1-4557-1122-2

Editor: Patrick Manley

Clinics in Podiatric Medicine and Surgery (ISSN 0891-8422) is published quarterly by Elsevier Inc., 360 Park Avenue South, New York, NY 10010-1710. Months of issue are January, April, July, and October. Business and Editorial Offices: 1600 John F. Kennedy Blvd., Ste. 1800, Philadelphia, PA 19103-2899. Customer Service Office: 3251 Riverport Lane, Maryland Heights, MO 63043. Periodicals postage paid at NewYork, NY and additional mailing offices. Subscription prices are $270.00 per year for US individuals, $385.00 per year for US institutions, $137.00 per year for US students and residents, $324.00 per year for Canadian individuals, $477.00 for Canadian institutions, $384.00 for international individuals, $477.00 per year for international institutions and $193.00 per year for Canadian and foreign students/residents. To receive student/resident rate, orders must be accompanied by name of affiliated institution, date of term, and the *signature* of program/residency coordinator on institution letterhead. Orders will be billed at individual rate until proof of status is received. Foreign air speed delivery is included in all *Clinics* subscription prices. All prices are subject to change without notice. POSTMASTER: Send address changes to *Clinics in Podiatric Medicine and Surgery*, Elsevier Health Sciences Division, Subscription Customer Service, 3251 Riverport Lane, Maryland Heights, MO 63043. **Customer Service: 1-800-654-2452 (US). From outside of the US, call 314-447-8871. Fax: 314-447-8029. E-mail: JournalsCustomerService-usa@elsevier.com (for print support); JournalsOnlineSupport-usa@elsevier.com (for online support).**

Reprints. For copies of 100 or more of articles in this publication, please contact the Commercial Reprints Department, Elsevier Inc., 360 Park Avenue South, New York, NY 10010-1710. Tel.: 212-633-3812; Fax: 212-462-1935; E-mail: reprints@elsevier.com.

Clinics in Podiatric Medicine and Surgery is covered in *MEDLINE/PubMed (Index Medicus)* and *EMBASE/Excerpta Medica.*

Printed and bound by CPI Group (UK) Ltd, Croydon, CR0 4YY

Transferred to Digital Print 2011

CLINICS IN PODIATRIC MEDICINE AND SURGERY

CONSULTING EDITOR
THOMAS ZGONIS, DPM, FACFAS

Contributors

CONSULTING EDITOR

THOMAS ZGONIS, DPM, FACFAS
Associate Professor, Reconstructive Foot and Ankle Fellowship Director and Chief,
Division of Podiatric Medicine and Surgery, Department of Orthopaedic Surgery,
University of Texas Health Science Center at San Antonio, San Antonio, Texas

GUEST EDITOR

PATRICK R. BURNS, DPM, FACFAS
Clinical Assistant Professor, Department of Orthopaedic Surgery, Division of Foot and
Ankle, University of Pittsburgh School of Medicine; Director, Podiatric Medicine and
Surgery Residency Program, University of Pittsburgh Medical Center, Pittsburgh,
Pennsylvania

AUTHORS

DAVID C. ALDER, DPM
Podiatry Residency Director, DeKalb Medical Center; Faculty, Podiatry Institute, Decatur,
Georgia

MICHELLE C. ANANIA, DPM
Ankle and Foot Care Centers, Youngstown, Ohio

GEORGE ANDROS, MD
Medical Director, Amputation Prevention Center, Valley Presbyterian Hospital,
Los Angeles, California

RONALD J. BELCZYK, DPM
Consultant Physician, Amputation Prevention Center, Valley Presbyterian Hospital,
Los Angeles, California

NICHOLAS J. BEVILACQUA, DPM, FACFAS
North Jersey Orthopaedic Specialists, Teaneck, New Jersey

PATRICK R. BURNS, DPM, FACFAS
Clinical Assistant Professor, Department of Orthopaedic Surgery, Division of Foot and
Ankle, University of Pittsburgh School of Medicine; Director, Podiatric Medicine and
Surgery Residency Program, University of Pittsburgh Medical Center, Pittsburgh,
Pennsylvania

BRANDON E. CRIM, DPM
University of Pittsburgh Medical Center, Pittsburgh, Pennsylvania

DEKARLOS M. DIAL, DPM
Cornerstone Foot and Ankle Specialists, High Point, North Carolina

LAWRENCE A. DIDOMENICO, DPM
Adjunct Professor, Ohio College of Podiatric Medicine; Director of Reconstructive
Rearfoot and Ankle Surgical Fellowship, Ankle and Foot Care Centers/Ohio College
of Podiatric Medicine; Chief, Section of Podiatric Medicine and Surgery, St Elizabeth's
Medical Center; Ankle and Foot Care Centers, Youngstown, Ohio

LESLIE B. DOWLING, DPM, MBA
Second Year Resident, DeKalb Medical Center, Decatur, Georgia

SPYRIDON P. GALANAKOS, MD, PhD
Department of Orthopaedics, General Hospital of Levadia, Levadia, Greece

ROBERT M. GREENHAGEN, DPM
Podiatric Surgeon, Private Practice, Foot and Ankle Center of Nebraska, Omaha,
Nebraska

GARY S. GRUEN, MD
Professor of Orthopaedic Surgery, Division of Orthopaedic Traumatology, Pittsburgh,
Pennsylvania

PETER HIGHLANDER, DPM, MS
Resident Physician, University of Pittsburgh Medical Center, Pittsburgh, Pennsylvania

ADAM R. JOHNSON, DPM
Podiatric Surgeon, Department of Surgery, Hennepin County Medical Center,
Minneapolis, Minnesota

ALISON JOSEPH, DPM
Attending Surgeon, University of Medicine and Dentistry of New Jersey, Newark,
New Jersey

CARL A. KIHM, DPM
Second Year Resident, DeKalb Medical Center, Decatur, Georgia

ANDREW J. KLUESNER, DPM, AACFAS
Foot and Ankle Surgeon, Department of Podiatric Medicine and Surgery, Christie Clinic,
Champaign, Illinois

NICHOLAS J. LOWERY, DPM
The Wound and Skin Healing Center at Washington Hospital, Washington, Pennsylvania

RYAN L. MCMILLEN, DPM
Orthopaedic Foot and Ankle Surgery Fellow, University of Pittsburgh Medical Center,
Pittsburgh, Pennsylvania

JARED L. MOON, DPM
Second Year Resident, DeKalb Medical Center, Decatur, Georgia

JASON B. MORRIS, DPM
Podiatric Foot and Ankle Specialist, University Foot and Ankle Institute, Foot and Ankle
Surgeon, Santa Barbara, California

VASSILIOS PAPATHANASIOU, MD
Department of Orthopaedics, General Hospital of Levadia, Levadia, Greece

DANIEL A. PEREZ, DPM
Second Year Resident, DeKalb Medical Center, Decatur, Georgia

LEE C. ROGERS, DPM
Associate Medical Director, Amputation Prevention Center, Valley Presbyterian Hospital, Los Angeles, California

MICHAEL RYAN, DPM
Cornerstone Foot and Ankle Specialists, High Point, North Carolina

IOANNIS P. SOFIANOS, MD
Department of Orthopaedics, General Hospital of Levadia, Levadia, Greece

JOHN J. STAPLETON, DPM, FACFAS
Associate, Foot and Ankle Surgery, VSAS Orthopaedics, Allentown; Clinical Assistant Professor of Surgery, Penn State College of Medicine, Hershey, Pennsylvania

TRAVIS STARK, BS
Research Assistant, Weil Foot and Ankle Institute, Des Plaines, Illinois

WENJAY SUNG, DPM
Fellowship-Trained Foot and Ankle Surgeon, Sinai Medical Group, Chicago, Illinois

LOWELL SCOTT WEIL Sr, DPM, FACFAS
Medical Director and CEO, Weil Foot and Ankle Institute, Des Plaines, Illinois

LOWELL WEIL Jr, DPM, MBA, FACFAS
Fellowship Director, Weil Foot and Ankle Institute, Des Plaines, Illinois

JASON B. WOODS, DPM
Resident, Podiatric Medicine and Surgery Program, University of Pittsburgh Medical Center, Pittsburgh, Pennsylvania

DANE K. WUKICH, MD
Chief, Division of Foot and Ankle; Assistant Residency Director; Associate Professor of Orthopaedic Surgery, University of Pittsburgh School of Medicine; Director, UPMC Comprehensive Foot and Ankle Center, Pittsburgh, Pennsylvania

Contents

> Internal fixation has become a pillar of surgical specialties, yet the evolution of these devices has been relatively short. The first known description of medical management of a fracture was found in the Edwin Smith Papyrus of Ancient Egypt (circa 2600 BC). The first description of internal fixation in the medical literature was in the 18th century. The advancement of techniques and technology over the last 150 years has helped to preserve both life and function. The pace of advancement continues to accelerate as surgeons continue to seek new technology for osseous fixation. The authors present a thorough review of the history of internal fixation and the transformation into a multibillion dollar industry.

> This article discusses the history of conventional plating, plate biomechanics, and screw function to provide better understanding of osseous physiology and biology using locking plates. The peer-reviewed and non–peer-reviewed literature have been researched to decipher and share the most pertinent information on this topic.

> Tibiotalocalcaneal arthrodesis for the treatment of complex foot and ankle deformities are extremely challenging cases. Technological advances in intramedullary nail fixation have improved the biomechanical properties of available fixation constructs in recent years. Nails designed specifically to accommodate hindfoot anatomy, advancement in the understanding of optimal screw orientation, fixed angle technology, the availability of spiral blade screws, and features designed to achieve compression across the arthrodesis site have provided the foot and ankle surgeon with a greater armamentarium for performing tibiotalocalneal arthrodesis. Although advances may help to improve clinical results, small sample sizes and the low-level evidence of study designs limit the evaluation of how these advances affect clinical outcomes.

Operative fixation of foot and ankle trauma can be challenging. Often times, the soft tissue envelope can have extensive damage as a result of the fracture. In these cases, percutaneous fixation may be used. Percutaneous fixation can benefit both soft tissue and osseous healing when used correctly. Many techniques have been described in the literature that may help to preserve blood supply, minimize soft tissue dissection, and restore a functional limb. This article reviews general guidelines for fracture and soft tissue management, osseous healing of fractures, and how certain techniques influence fracture healing. It also illustrates certain techniques for specific fracture reduction.

One of the most widely debated topics amongst foot and ankle surgeons is the treatment of end stage arthritis. With the advent of the newer generation of total ankle replacement (TAR), a viable option over an arthrodesis is now available for patients with end-stage ankle arthritis. When compared with an ankle arthroplasty, recent reports suggest the ankle arthrodesis has poor long-term outcomes (20 years+) and can experience short- and long-term complications. Proper training, strict patient selection, and proper implant contribute to a successful outcome. As advances continue to be made in both implant design and surgical technique, the benefits of a TAR appears to provide the foot and ankle surgeon a good alternative for the appropriate patient.

Arthroereisis has gained popularity over the years because it eliminates excessive pronation while conserving preoperative inversion and preserves forefoot to rearfoot adaptation to uneven terain. Technically simple, some of the advantages of subtalar arthroereisis are that it is joint sparing and preserves ligaments. In addition, the implant does not interfere with osseous growth and does not compromise future operative intervention if more invasive procedures are required. Arthroereisis, however, can have associated complications along with the need for surgical removal in some patient populations.

The first metatarsophalangeal (MTP) joint is a frequent diseased-affected articulation encountered by the foot and ankle surgeon. Arthroplasty remains a favorable option for surgeons, because it preserves motion of the joint. The authors' focus at the Weil Foot and Ankle Institute has been on using double-stem silicone implants with titanium grommets, which may be a viable solution for affected articulations. The authors present their clinical

FORTHCOMING ISSUES

RECENT ISSUES

THE CLINICS ARE NOW AVAILABLE ONLINE!

Access your subscription at:
www.theclinics.com

Foreword

Advances in Fixation Technology for the Foot and Ankle

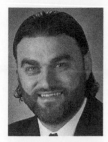

Thomas Zgonis, DPM
Consulting Editor

The evolution to the current technology of internal and external fixation for the foot and ankle is simply fascinating. As I look back over the last decade, it is amazing to follow the progression of how some of the surgical procedure performances and selections have changed. Advances in fixation technology for the foot and ankle are simply evident by the seemingly endless stream of new products within the field of foot and ankle surgery. This edition of *Clinics in Podiatric Medicine and Surgery* is able to incorporate the most recent advances in technology that have helped foot and ankle surgeons to manage some of the most challenging clinical case scenarios.

The guest editor, Dr Burns, and his colleagues were chosen for their surgical expertise and knowledge and to overview concisely a vast array of fixation methods that are currently available. In addition, possible complications with these novel techniques and products are also discussed. I thank all the authors for a job well done, as the articles are exciting to read and provide thoughtful insight to the management of complex foot and ankle conditions.

Thomas Zgonis, DPM
Division of Podiatric Medicine and Surgery
Department of Orthopaedic Surgery
University of Texas Health Science Center at San Antonio
7703 Floyd Curl Drive – MSC 7776
San Antonio, TX 78229, USA

E-mail address:
zgonis@uthscsa.edu

Clin Podiatr Med Surg 28 (2011) xv
doi:10.1016/j.cpm.2011.08.006
0891-8422/11/$ – see front matter © 2011 Elsevier Inc. All rights reserved.

podiatric.theclinics.com

Preface

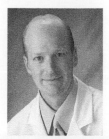

Patrick R. Burns, DPM
Guest Editor

I am proud to be guest editor of this edition and present to you a review of the evolution in fixation as it relates to the foot and ankle. Over the last ten years, there has been tremendous growth in our field and evidence-based medicine is helping to drive our knowledge and outcomes. This is an exciting time with advancements in fixation allowing us to increase our abilities and indications.

Fixation techniques have always been important but in years past sometimes difficult due to the complexity of size, shape, and mechanics of a weight-bearing lower extremity. With the increasing skill of surgeons and the drive to continue to improve, there has been a need for advancements in fixation. Increasing knowledge in fixation mechanics and principles along with improvements in materials and design have produced significant growth in the foot and ankle surgeon's armamentarium.

There are now many choices in fixation and this edition is to be used as an informative guide. Articles cover topics such as locking plate technology, anatomic-shaped designs, percutaneous applications, fixation in patients with complicated diabetes, and newer uses of external fixation. There is a balance, however, and these improvements must be used conscientiously. Technology comes at a price and needs to be recognized. But, with the proper knowledge of indications and applications, these new technologies will continue our growth and ultimately patient outcomes.

Patrick R. Burns, DPM
Division of Foot and Ankle
University of Pittsburgh Medical Center
Roesch Taylor Building
2100 Jane Street, Suite 7100
Pittsburgh, PA 15203, USA

E-mail address:
burnsp@upmc.edu

doi:10.1016/j.cpm.2011.08.007
0891-8422/11/$ – see front matter © 2011 Elsevier Inc. All rights reserved.
podiatric.theclinics.com

Internal Fixation: a Historical Review

Robert M. Greenhagen, DPM[a],*, Adam R. Johnson, DPM[b],
Alison Joseph, DPM[c]

KEYWORDS

• Historical review • Internal fixation • AO • Foot ankle surgery

HISTORICAL OVERVIEW OF INTERNAL FIXATION

Internal fixation has become a pillar of surgical specialties, yet the evolution of these devices has been relatively short. The first known description of medical management of a fracture was found in the Edwin Smith Papyrus of Ancient Egypt (circa 2600 BC).[1] The medical text described the use of a splint and bandaging with honey, grease, and lint for a humeral fracture.[1] This technique of splintage and bandaging was further advanced by Hippocrates[2] and remained the dominant treatment protocol for 4000 years. The advancement of techniques and technology over the last 150 years has helped to preserve both life and function. The pace of advancement continues to accelerate as surgeons continue to seek new technology for osseous fixation.

Some early civilizations using internal fixation were reported by explorers and ambassadors to these lands.[3,4] Reports of intramedullary (IM) devices are seen in Egyptian, Aztec, and Inca societies,[3–5] whereas in Europe, even at the end of the eighteenth century, the use of internal fixation remained controversial. One of the earliest recorded uses of internal fixation is one of accusation and controversy. In 1775, in a prominent French surgical journal 1 surgeon accused others of having caused the death of a patient by inserting brass wire to fix a humeral fracture[6,7]:

To hold the fracture fragments in position, without need for any difficult and awkward dressing, made deep, longitudinal incisions in the soft tissue and introduced immediately around the bone, piercing the flesh, brass wires, which he made into several rings; he encircled the bone fragments in these rings somewhat crudely and he carefully twisted the ends around each other. This beautiful maneuver had the expected result: inflammation and gangrene from which the patient died 2 days later.[7]

The accused surgeon, Jean Francois Icart, responded by denying the event, but stated that this technique was commonly used by 2 well-known surgeons, F. Lapeyode and M. Sicre of Toulouse, France.[7,8] Therefore, these 2 surgeons have been credited with the first use of internal fixation in modern times.[9]

[a] Private Practice, Foot and Ankle Center of Nebraska, Omaha, NE, USA
[b] Department of Surgery, Hennepin County Medical Center, Minneapolis, MN, USA
[c] University of Medicine and Dentistry of New Jersey, Newark, NJ, USA
* Corresponding author.
E-mail address: robert.m.greenhagen@gmail.com

Clin Podiatr Med Surg 28 (2011) 607–618
doi:10.1016/j.cpm.2011.06.006
0891-8422/11/$ – see front matter © 2011 Elsevier Inc. All rights reserved.

The delay in advancement of internal fixation was caused by a lack of adjunct technology. A necessary continuum of medical discoveries was required to create an environment of routine and successful internal fixation. These discoveries include anesthesia by William Thomas Green Morton in 1846,[10] antisepsis by Joseph Lister in 1867,[11] the invention of radiographs in 1895 by Wilhelm Conrad Röntgen,[12] and Sir Alexander Fleming's discovery of penicillin in 1928.[13]

In 1958, 4 prominent Swiss surgeons, Martin Allgöwer, Maurice E. Müller, Robert Schneider, and Hans Willenegger, founded the Arbeitsgemeinschaft für Osteosynthesefragen (AO) (the Association for the Study of Internal Fixation [ASIF]). These pioneers believed that the treatment of fractures can be improved by means of surgical procedures and internal fixation with implants. They forged a strategic alliance with Mathys Medizinaltechnik, a company active in Swiss precision engineering, to develop and produce an integrated system of implants and instruments.

The first undertaking by the foundation was the establishment of the Laboratory for Experimental Surgery (Forschungsinstitut) in Davos, Switzerland by Martin Allgöwer with the appointment of Herbert Fleisch as the director in 1963. The early work that was conducted, together with that of Schenk and Willenegger, laid the groundwork for the current knowledge of direct and indirect fracture healing, as well as the influence of rigid fixation on the healing of delayed and nonunions. Their classic landmark experiments are known to fracture surgeons throughout the world. The early AO pioneers also forged a strategic alliance with the Swiss precision engineering discipline and worked closely with Robert Mathys and Fritz Straumann to develop an integrated system of implants and instrumentation for fracture fixation. The developed instrumentation and implant devices would enable surgical fracture fixations to fulfill the biomechanical principles devised after years of experimental work. This fruitful collaboration led to the evolution of the AO instrumentation and their corresponding surgical techniques. The final piece was to document carefully their surgical cases. The Documentation Center that was created allowed continuing education of their emerging technology.[14]

Advances in Metallurgy

Implant material plays a vital role in the success of internal fixation. The study of metallurgy in internal fixation started with H.S. Levert's work in 1829. Levert studied gold, silver, lead, and platinum in vivo in an attempt to understand the biocompatibility of each metal.[15] From that time, the oldest implants for internal fixation of fractures were made from various materials, including ivory, bone, and metals of bronze, lead, gold, copper, silver, brass, steel, and aluminum alloys. This material was observed in steel-pointed silver pins in wounds. Ivory and bone pegs were used most commonly for IM fixation in early fracture treatment. Based on German research these materials were shown to reabsorb into the body without reactions like early metals, yielding fewer infections and nonunions.[16–19] Nicholas Senn, an American surgeon, worked extensively on the use of ivory and bone in fracture fixation and developed a hollow perforated intraosseous splint, as well as an extramedullary sleeve from ox bone that absorbed in the body as the fracture healed.[20] Because of his pioneering work, Nicholas Senn can be called the father of biodegradable implants.[21]

Silver was common early in the evolution of fixation, and often used for cerclage wires, plates, and IM pins. The use of silver wire was first reported by John Kearney-Rogers, an American surgeon, in 1827.[22] In 1838, Achille-Cléophas Flaubert, reported by his assistant Laloy, reportedly used silver wire for the reduction of an open humeral fracture.[23] Elias Samuel Cooper was the first to combine internal fixation with antisepsis in 1861, when he used silver wire and alcohol for the fixation of acromioclavicular joint injuries.[24] In 1877, Lister performed osteosynthesis of a closed fracture of the patella, under carbolic acid spray, using a silver wire.[25]

The first constructed plates were made from nickel-coated sheet steel, silver, aluminum, and brass,[26–29] William O'Neil Sherman, a surgeon for the Carnegie Steel Company in Pittsburgh, Pennsylvania, introduced vanadium steel and self-tapping screws in 1912.[27] Nevertheless, all the metals were highly problematic from the viewpoint of their mechanical properties, corrosion, and incompatibility with living tissue. The problems that plagued the early implants were eventually resolved with the advent and use of stainless steel. Although stainless steel was invented before the First World War, it was not used for the production of implants until 1931.[30] The use of stainless steel proved to be the first significant breakthrough in the development of internal fixation. The excellent corrosion-resistant property, strength, and biocompatibility of stainless steel have kept it in use even to modern times with only slight modifications. Surgical grade stainless alloys (316L) are made with a combination of iron, chromium, and nickel. The low carbon (L) in the steel diminishes corrosion and adverse tissue reactions and allergies.

Metallic implants saw further advancement when Charles Scott Venable and Walter Goodloe Stuck introduced the cobalt alloy in 1936[31] and in 1951, when a titanium alloy was promoted by Gottlieb Leventhal.[32] Stainless steel has been a mainstay for plates, screws, and IM devices that do not provide extended weight bearing, but because this metal is prone to fatigue failure and has a high corrosion rate it is a poor candidate for the manufacturing of modern joint replacement implants.[33] Alloys made of cobalt, chromium, and molybdenum can be created to have varying porous forms, allowing ingrown and biologic fixation and are well suited for the production of surgical implants that are required to be load bearing. Cobalt alloys were used in the first generation of joint replacement implants and are still commonly used. Titanium also has a high level of biocompatibility along with a low level of corrosion. Titanium is used in many implants and has garnered excellent long-term results. Although titanium materials have been used successfully worldwide for many years, there is controversy within the medical community about reactions to the metal placed within the body during surgery: some patients develop skin reactions and wound infections, necessitating presurgery testing for metal sensitivity.

The 1959 discovery of Nitinol (named after the Nickel-Titanium Naval Ordnance Laboratory) by William J. Buehler was praised for providing fatigue resistance of the metal.[34] Nitinol is most commonly known for its mechanical or shape-memory property, which refers to the ability of the metal to undergo deformation at 1 temperature, then recover its original shape when heated. This characteristic of this metal was not discovered until 1961, when during a presentation of the metal David S. Muzzey, who was a pipe smoker, applied his pipe lighter to compress the sample metal strand and noted its curious effect.[35] However, by the 1970, problems with corrosion were being seen in those with the stainless devices.

Researchers are continually developing new materials for use in internal fixation for orthopaedic surgery. Currently research is being conducted on the metal tantalum, which is remarkably resistant to corrosion and has been used as an ingredient to create superalloys. Tantalum been applied to the manufacturing of implants and research has been promising.[36,37]

Another area of recent interest has been the development of biomaterials. These materials are not only compatible with tissues of the body but many reabsorb or dissolve after the bone has healed. Current materials in this field being researched and beginning to be used as implants are poly-L-lactic acid (PLLA), polyether-etherketone (PEEK), and hydroxylapatite.

Advances in Design

Research and innovation have facilitated advances in fixation technique and design. The earliest documented fixation designs are simple, beginning with examples such as cerclage wire. Newer ideas generally rose from complications along with the increased understanding of the mechanics of the injury and repair.

Cerclage wire, pins, and staples

As mentioned earlier, the first report of internal fixation involved wiring of long bone fractures by F. Lapujode and M. Sicre around 1760.[9] In 1912 a surgeon by the name of Robert Milne described a modified technique in which flexible pins could be used in cerclage fashion.[38] A modification of this technique used narrow bands of metal and was described by 2 separate investigators, Italian surgeon Vittorio Putti and American surgeon Frederick William Parham. These implants would later be named Putti-Parham bands and had limited applications.[39,40] This limitation was most likely because of the need for extensive dissection that achieved only minimal stabilization. Cerclage wire remains a viable option but has limited applications. In foot and ankle surgery, it is generally used in tension banding of medial malleolar and fifth metatarsal base fractures.

The use of simple pin fixation began with advent of skeletal traction and external fixation. The first documented fixation by use of pins was described by Paul Neihans in 1904.[41] In 1908, Fritz Steinmann published his results of pin fixation for the use of traction and external fixation,[42] but this was not the first description of the technique: Italian orthopaedist Alessandro Codivilla had described a similar means of applying traction in 1903[43] and later publicly accused Steinmann of stealing his idea. Martin Kirschner introduced his thinner traction pin in 1909.[44] The use of pin fixation was popularized by Lorenz Böhler, the father of modern trauma, in his groundbreaking text *Technik der Knochenbruchbehandlung* (*The Treatment of Fractures*) in 1929. Forms of simple pin fixation are still used in external fixation, guide wires for cannulated screws, pinning across physeal plates, tension band technique, and others.

As an extension of the simple pin, staples were created. Alberto Jacocel first described the use of osseous staple fixation in 1901.[41] In foot and ankle surgery, staples continue to have various uses such as phalangeal osteotomies, calcaneal osteotomies, and midfoot fusions. Recently, significant changes to the simple staple have included the integration of memory metals, manual compression designs, and variable staple leg lengths and angles.

IM Nail

IM nailing was the first consistently performed procedure in which internal fixation was used. Bernardino de Sahagun, a sixteenth century anthropologist who traveled to Mexico with Hernando Cortes, reported the use of IM wooden pegs by Aztec and Inca civilizations for the treatment of long bone nonunions.[3,4] In 1995, scientists from Brigham Young University found evidence of advanced internal fixation in an Egyptian sarcophagus with the name Usermontu, although the mummy is not believed to be the high priest Usermontu, so the age of the mummy is also unknown (**Fig. 1**).[5] It is also unclear if the device was placed while the person was living or just before mummification. What is clear is this advanced design and surgical technique were unmatched for thousands of years.

The first record of IM nailing in modern medical literature was in 1846 by German surgeon J.F. Dieffenbach.[19] In 1850, Benhard von Langenbeck became the first surgeon to use internal fixation after a surgically created osteotomy. He inserted an ivory IM device into a patient's mandible.[45] The first to describe an IM device (made

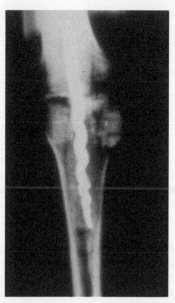

Fig. 1. Intramedullary device discovered in the knee of a mummy in Rosicrucian Egyptian Museum. The device was inserted post-humorously prior to the mummification process and made of iron. (Photograph courtesy of and copyright to Rosicrucian Egyptian Museum, San Jose, CA.)

of ivory) for acute fracture fixation was H. Bircher in 1887.[46] In 1890, Themistocles Gluck increased the stability of these ivory devices by introducing an interlocked IM design. Metal used for IM fixation was introduced in 1914, when Ernest Hey Groves described 3 cases of metallic IM nailing for gunshot wounds.[47,48] This material did not gain momentum early on because of a high rate of infection, which gave Groves the nickname Septic Ernie.

Early on, surgeons still preferred their IM devices to be made of ivory. Unlike other early materials, ivory resorbs. In contrast, it was believed the body would react to metals, creating a fibrotic nest around the material, increasing rates of nonunion, dehiscence, and infection.[16,17] However, all of this changed when Marius Nygaard Smith-Petersen had success with the use of stainless steel IM nails in 1931, and a shift to using the metal began.[49] In the United States, brothers Leslie Vaughn and Hubery Lowry Rush became the first American surgeons to use IM fixation. In 1939 the material was modified to pins named Rush pins or Rush rods, which gained popularity.[50] The German-born Gerhard Küntscher, whom many consider the father of modern IM techniques, reported the principle of elastic union, in which the IM device acts as an internal splint within the medullary canal.[51] Küntscher's work gained some interest while he was working with Smith-Petersen but his early work was not well received in Germany by the traditional orthopaedic hierarchy.[3] With little seniority, he was sent to the northern Finnish front during World War II, but continued his work.[3] At the end of the War, the world began to notice the advancements that Küntscher was making with his fixation technique. Although he is not the first to describe the use of IM fixation for the treatment of acute lower extremity fractures, Küntscher is the single most important individual for the advancement of IM fixation. Important contributions included immediate mobilization after IM nailing and the use of IM reaming. Küntscher was also the first surgeon to describe the use of IM fixation for tibiotalocalcaneal fusions.[52]

In modern foot and ankle surgery, intermedullary devices are most commonly used for the treatment of tibial fractures and hindfoot fusions. For some surgeons Rush rod/pins are still used for transverse fibular fractures; newer devices are gaining popularity such as the bolt technique for midfoot Charcot neuroarthropathy reconstruction.

Screws and Plate

The first use of screw fixation began with the advent of external fixation. As surgical techniques advanced, these devices became an internal form of fixation. Rigaud of Strasbourg is credited with the first use of screw fixation for fracture fixation. In 1850, Rigaud used 2 screws for the reduction of a displaced olecranon fracture.[53] From the description, he may also be the first surgeon to have used the tension band technique.[53]

Once the use of osseous screws was established, this allowed the advent of plate fixation. The first published report of successful plate fixation was the results of Carl Hansmann of Germany in 1886 using a flat plate made of an alloy of nickel, copper, and tin with unicortical screws that were drilled through and locked into the plate.[26] The first complete implantation of plate and screws for fixation was performed by William Stewart Halsted in 1893 using a plate made of silver.[54,55] In 1894 William Arbuthnot Lane was credited with the implantation of a steel plate. The plate that Lane used was flat and the screws were designed with a lag in the treads and were the precursor of current cancellous thread forms.[54] Flat plates had their obvious inherited faults and it did not take long for Albin Lamotte in the early 1900s to advocate curving plates transversely to better fit the curved bone as well as a narrower, fully threaded screw, which evolved into the current cortical thread forms.[54] Another advancement to the use of plate and screw fixation occurred in 1915, when William O'Neil Sherman, a surgeon for the Carnegie Steel Company in Pittsburgh, introduced a self-tapping screw.[41] English surgeon Earnest Hey Groves studied the early work of Lane, noting loosening of the screw fixation.[56] Hey Groves recognized a traditional wood screw design was inappropriate for bone because of the dense homogenous makeup; furthermore, he recognized the advantages of the engineering screw described by Lambotte and the self-tapping slit by Sherman.[56] In 1956 George Bagby developed the first dynamic compression plate with offset screw holes that created compression on the fracture site once placed.[57] In 1988, Perren and colleagues[58,59] showed the osseous-plate interface leads to local necrosis and later developed a plate that had limited contact with the osseous interface and provided compression. In 1916 Hey Groves was credited with describing the first locking plate design in which the heads of the screws screwed directly into the plate construct.[60] Paul Reinhold, a French surgeon, patented a similar plate design to Hey Groves in 1931, and it was commercialized in 1935.[54] Locking plates later reemerged in Europe with the Wolter system in 1974 and the Zespol System in 1982.[61,62]

Plates and screws continue to be some of the most popular devices in foot and ankle surgery. Plating systems have become more anatomically specific for the unique architecture of the foot, and specialty plates such as those that include an opening wedge are improving technique.

Further technological improvements such as locking plates are also improving outcomes in patients at high risk, such as those with diabetes and osteoporosis. These evolutions are part of the expanding market in orthopaedic implantable devices.

Box 1 Overall sales 2009	
Company	Sales ($)
Stryker Corp	6.7 billion
DePuy Orthopaedics (J&J)	5.4 billion
Zimmer Holdings	4.1 billion
Smith & Nephew	3.8 billion
Medtronic Spinal & Biologics	3.4 billion
Synthes	3.4 billion
Biomet	2.5 billion
DJO Inc.	946 million
Orthofix	546 million
Wright Medical	488 million

Data from Delporte C, Barbella M. The top 10. ODT. 2010 ed. Ramsey (NJ): Rodman Publishing, 2010.

Advances on an Industry

The age of the medical device industry established itself when Thomas Codman introduced his Ether Pocket Cupping Instrument in the 1830s in Boston, Massachusetts.[63] In 1895 the first commercial orthopaedic manufacturer in the world was established when DePuy was founded by Revra DePuy in Warsaw, Indiana. DePuy's goal was to provide a fiber splint to replace the wooden barrel staves then used to set fractures.[63] Further growth in the industry occurred in 1927, when Raymond Zimmer and surgeon C.F. Lytle produced a series of 50 aluminum splints and presented them at the American Medical Association meeting that year. Other devices followed for Zimmer, and in the first year the business earned $160,000.[64] 1941 marks the year when the Stryker Corporation was established by Homer Stryker to create more innovative medical equipment, such as the cast cutting saw.[65] Wright Manufacturing entered the market in 1950 after founder Frank O. Wright noted that individuals in leg casts were prone to chronic back pain from walking on the hard steel heel in the foot of the cast. To alleviate this situation, Wright developed a rubber heel to provide shock absorption and decrease the impact while walking, marketing the device as the Street Heel.[66]

Eventually the founders of fixation principles noted the lucrative endeavor present and joined into the frenzy in 1960. AO/ASIF formed an industrial cooperation with the Straumann Institute to produce implants under the trademarked name of Synthes and held the rights for its intellectual property. In 2006, the implant subsidiary had become so successful that Synthes acquired the Synthes trade name and trademarks

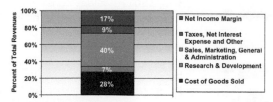

Fig. 2. Where does it go? Estimated percentage of expenditures per implanted device. (*From* FY 2004 10K reports for Stryker, Smith and Nephew, Zimmer, Wright Medical, Encore Medical, Exatech. Medtronic figures are from the 4 consecutive quarters ending January 28, 2005. Biomet figures are from 4 consecutive quarters ending in February 28, 2005.)

Box 2	
Extremity sales 2009 (with estimated fourth quarter)	
Company	Sales ($ million)
DePuy	235.5
Tornier	157.5
Zimmer	133.6
Wright Medical	106.4
Biomet	85.6
ArthroCare	68.5
Ascension Orthopedics	24.2
Exactech	22.9
Stryker	22.4
Others	180.4

Data from Joshi D. Extremity market aims for $1billion. Orthopedics this week. Wayne (PA): RRY Publications, 2009.

as well as all intellectually property from the AO Foundation to become its own corporation.[67]

Soon many companies entered the market, each providing unique products and continuing the innovation of a growing industry. Despite such high levels of competition in the medical implant industry, the top 15 companies accounted for 95% of the market share in 2009 (**Box 1**). The top 5 companies were responsible for more than 60% of $37.8 billion sales in 2009.[68–70] Sales have continued to increase for orthopaedic devices, with an overall growth rate of 6.2% in 2009.[69] These companies continue to research new technology, although research spending remains less than the 10% of most company's expenditures (**Fig. 2**). However, the new devices produced are double edged. New technology and designs may aid in outcomes,

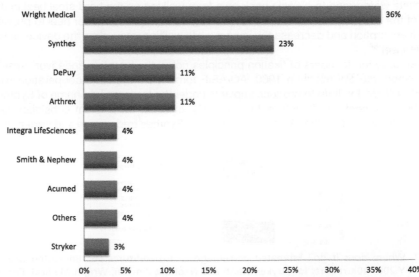

Fig. 3. Leading company in foot and ankle surgical devices. (*Data from* Joshi D. What do the foot and ankle surgeons have to say. Fort Wayne (IN): PeralDiver Technologies; 2008.)

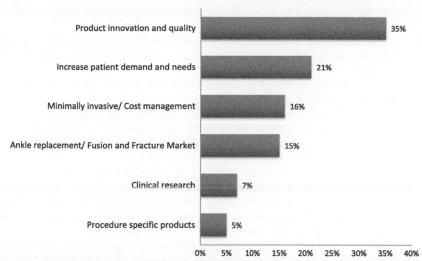

Fig. 4. Most important factor when choosing a device. (*Data from* Joshi D. What do the foot and ankle surgeons have to say. Fort Wayne (IN): PeralDiver Technologies, 2008.)

but may be disruptive because continued high costs of newer implants may affect insurance cost and reimbursement.

The market for extremities, which includes foot and ankle devices, is a small yet fast-growing sector of orthopaedics. Sales reached $1 billion in 2009, with a growth rate of 14%.[71] Extremities device sales have been rising steeply over the past decade and grew by more than 110% between 2005 and 2008.[71] Because the market is relatively new it remains competitive. The top 5 companies (DePuy, Wright Medical, Tornier, Zimmer, and Biomet) make up 70% of the total extremity market (**Box 2**). When foot and ankle surgeons were surveyed Wright Medical and Synthes were perceived as the best companies (**Fig. 3**)[72]; in addition, the most important factor was product innovation and quality (**Fig. 4**).[72]

SUMMARY

Although the evolution of internal fixation is short, it has been dynamic. From the first reports in the late eighteenth century to the multibillion dollar industry today, we have striven to improve our techniques and materials in the hope of better outcomes. In the near future, the increasing costs may have a profound effect on the developing technology because cost controls must be initiated to prevent the collapse of the industry.

REFERENCES

1. Breasted JH. The Edwin Smith surgical papyrus. Chicago: University of Chicago Press; 1930.
2. Hippocrates Adams F. The genuine works of Hippocrates. London: Sydenham Society; 1849.
3. Bong MR, Koval KJ, Egol KA. The history of intramedullary nailing. Bull NYU Hosp Jt Dis 2006;64:94–7.
4. Knothe U, Knothe Tate ML, Perren SM. 300 years of intramedullary fixation–from Aztec practice to standard treatment modality. Eur J Trauma 2000;26:217–25.

5. Snow K. BYU professor finds evidence of advanced surgery in ancient mummy. Provo (UT): BYU Magazine; 1996.
6. Pujol A. Mèmoire sur une amputation naturelle de la jambe avec des rèflexions sur quelques autres cas relatifs à l'amputation. J Med Chir Pharm (Paris) 1775; 160 [in German].
7. Evans PE. Cerclage fixation of a fractured humerus in 1775. Fact or fiction? Clin Orthop Relat Res 1983;174:138–42.
8. Icart JF. Lettre à reponse au mèmoire de M Pujol, mèdecin et de l'hôtel-dieu, sur une amputation naturelle de la jambe avec des reflexions sur quelques autres cas relatifs à cette opèration. J Med Chir Pharm (Paris) 1775;164 [in French].
9. Guthrie G. Direct fixation in fractures. Am Med 1903;376.
10. Morton WT. Remarks on the proper mode of administering sulphuric ether by inhalation. Boston: Button and Wentworth; 1847.
11. Lister J. On the antiseptic principle in the practice of surgery. Br Med J 1867;2:246–8.
12. Röntgen WC. Über eine neue Art von Strahlen. Vorläufige Mitteilung. Sitzungsberichte der Würzburger physik-medic 1895;137–47 [in German].
13. Fleming A. On the antibacterial action of cultures of a penicillium, with special reference to their use in the isolation of *B. influenzae*. Br J Exp Pathol 1929;10: 226–36.
14. History. AO Foundation. Switzerland: AO Publishing; 2010.
15. Ratner BD, Hoffman AS, Schoen FJ, et al. Biomaterials science: an introduction to materials in medicine. 2nd edition. San Diego (CA): Elsevier; 2004.
16. Konig F. Uber die Implantation von Elfenbein zum Ersatz von Knochen und Gelenken. Nach Experimentellen und klinischen Beobachtungen. Beitr Klin Chir 1913;91–114 [in German].
17. Bircher H. Eine neue Methode unmittelbarer Retention bei Fracturen der Rohrenknochen. Arch Klin Chir 1886;410–22 [in German].
18. Aufrecht E. Ueber riesenzellen in Elfenbeinstiften, welche zur Heilung einer Pseudoarthrose eingekeilt waren. Centrallblat Med Wissensch 1877;465–7 [in German].
19. Dieffenbach JF. Neue sichere Heilmethode des falschen Gelenkes oder der Pseudoarthrose mittels Durchbohrung der Knochen und einschlagen von Zappfen. Casper's Wochenschriftt Gesam Heilk 1846;727–34, 745–52, 761–5 [in German].
20. Senn N. A new method of direct fixation of the fragments in compound and ununited fractures. Ann Surg 1893;18(2):125–51.
21. Bartonicek J. Early history of operative treatment of fractures. Arch Orthop Trauma Surg 2010;130:1385–96.
22. Rodgers J. Case of ununited fracture of the os brachii successfully treated. New York Med Phys J 1927;6:521–3.
23. Laloy LH. De la suture des os appliqueè aux resections et aux fractures avec plaie. Paris: Rignoux; 1839.
24. Cooper ES. New method of treating long standing dislocations of the scapuloclavicular articulation. Am J Med Sci 1861;41:389–92.
25. Lister J. An address on the treatment of fracture of the patella. Br Med J 1883;2: 855–60.
26. Hansmann C. Eine neue Methode der Fixierung der Fragmente bei komplizierten Frakturen. Verh Dtsch Ges Chir 1886;14:134–7 [in German].
27. Sherman WO. Vanadium steel bone plates ad screws. Surg Gyn Obst 1912;629–34.
28. Steinbach LW. IV. On the use of fixation plates in the treatment of fractures of the leg. Ann Surg 1900;31:436–42.

29. Blake JA. The operative treatment of fractures. Surg Gyn Obst 1912;43(14): 338–45.
30. Venable CS, Stuck WG. The internal fixation of fractures. Oxford (UK): Blackwell Scientific Publications; 1947.
31. Venable CS, Stuck WG, Beach A. The effects on bone of the presence of metals; based upon electrolysis: an experimental study. Ann Surg 1937;105:917–38.
32. Leventhal GS. Titanium, a metal for surgery. J Bone Joint Surg Am 1951;33: 473–4.
33. Yoo YR, Jang SG, Oh KT, et al. Influences of passivating elements on the corrosion and biocompatibility of super stainless steels. J Biomed Mater Res B Appl Biomater 2008;86:310–20.
34. Buehler WJ, Gilfrich JW, Wiley RC. Effects of low-temperature phase changes on the mechanical properties of alloys near composition tini. J Appl Phys 1963;34: 1475–7.
35. Kauffman GB, Mayo I. The story of Nitinol: the serendipitous discovery of the memory metal and its applications. The Chemical Educator 1997;2: 1–21.
36. Harrison AK, Gioe TJ, Simonelli C, et al. Do porous tantalum implants help preserve bone? evaluation of tibial bone density surrounding tantalum tibial implants in TKA. Clin Orthop Relat Res 2010;468:2739–45.
37. Levine B, Sporer S, Della Valle CJ, et al. Porous tantalum in reconstructive surgery of the knee: a review. J Knee Surg 2007;20:185–94.
38. Milne R. Remarks. Clin JB Murphy 1913;38:229–34.
39. Parham FW. Circular constriction in the treatment of fractures of the long bones. Surg Gyn Obst 1916;23:541–4.
40. Putti V. Un nuovo metodo di osteosintesi. Clin Chir 1914;22:1021–4.
41. Peltier LF. Fractures: a history and iconography of their treatment. San Francisco (CA): Norman Publishing; 1990.
42. Steinmann F. Eine neue Extensionsmethode in der Frakturbehandlung. Zentralbl Chir 1907;34:153–6 [in German].
43. Codivilla A. Sulla correzione della deformita de frattura del femore. Bull Sci Med (Bologna) 1903;3:246–9 [in Italian].
44. Kirschner M. Ueber Nagelextension. Beitr Klin Chir 1909;64:266 [in German].
45. Contzen H. Development of intramedullary nailing and the interlocking nail. Aktuelle Traumatol 1987;17:250–2 [in German].
46. Bircher H. Eine neue Methode unmittelbarer Retention bei Fracturen der Röhrenknochen. Arch Klin Chir 1887;410–22 [in German].
47. Hey Groves EW. On the application of the principle of extension to comminuted fractures of the long bone, with special reference to gunshot injuries. Br J Surg 1914;2:429–43.
48. Gluck T. Autoplastic transplantation, implantation von Fremdkorpern. Berliner Kliische Wochenschrift 1881;18:529.
49. Smith-Petersen MN. Intracapsular fractures of the neck of the femur. Treatment by internal fixation. Arch Surg 1931;64:715–59.
50. Rush LV, Rush HL. A reconstruction operation for a comminuted fracture of the upper third of the ulna. Am J Surg 1937;38:332–3.
51. Küntscher G. Die Marknalung von Knochenbruchen. Langenbecks Arch Klin Chir 1940;200:443–55 [in German].
52. Küntscher G. Praxis der Marknagelung. Stuttgart (Germany): Schattauer; 1962.
53. Cucuel LR, Rigaud R. Des vis métalliques enfoncees dans le tissue des os. Pour le traitment de certaines fractures. Revue Med Chir Paris 1850;8:113–5 [in French].

54. Russell TA. An historical perspective of the development of plate and screw fixation and minimally invasive fracture surgery with a unified biological approach. Techniques in Orthopaedics 2007;22:186–90.
55. Lathan SR. Dr. Halsted at Hopkins and at High Hampton. Proc (Bayl Univ Med Cent) 2010;23:33–7.
56. Hey Groves EW. On modern methods of treating fractures. 2nd edition. Bristol (United Kingdom): John Wright; 1921.
57. Bagby GW, Janes JM. The effect of compression on the rate of fracture healing using a special plate. Am J Surg 1958;95:761–71.
58. Stannard JP, Schmidt AH, Kregor PJ. Surgical treatment of orthopaedic trauma. New York: Thieme; 2007.
59. Perren SM, Cordey J, Rahn BA, et al. Early temporary porosis of bone induced by internal fixation implants. A reaction to necrosis, not to stress protection? Clin Orthop Relat Res 1988;232:139–51.
60. Hey Groves EW. On modern methods of treating fractures. Bristol (United Kingdom): John Wright; 1916.
61. Wolter. Innovative locking plate system. 1992. US Patent 5085660.
62. Ramotowski W, Granowski R. Zespol. An original method of stable osteosynthesis. Clin Orthop Relat Res 1991;272:67–75.
63. Depuy: history. Available at: http://www.depuy.com/about-depuy/corporate-info/history. Accessed October 14, 2010.
64. Zimmer history–milestones 1900–1930. Zimmer; 2010. Available at: http://www.zimmer.com/z/ctl/op/global/action/1/id/10161/template/CP/navid/10098. Accessed October 14, 2010.
65. Stryker–about us– history. Stryker Corporation; 2010. Available at: http://www.trauma.stryker.com/general/history.php?tab=0&vis=pts&loc=asi. Accessed October 14, 2010.
66. Company history. Wright Medical Group; 2010. Available at: http://www.fundinguniverse.com/company-histories/Wright-Medical-Group-Inc-Company-History.html. Accessed October 14, 2010.
67. Armstrong DG, Lavery LA, Kimbriel HR, et al. Activity patterns of patients with diabetic foot ulceration: patients with active ulceration may not adhere to a standard pressure off-loading regimen. Diabetes Care 2003;26:2595–7.
68. Delporte C, Barbella M. The top 10. ODT. 2010. Ramsey (NJ): Rodman Publishing; 2010.
69. The 2009–2010 orthopaedic industry annual report. Chagrin Falls (OH): OrthoWorld; 2010.
70. Young R. 2010: through a glass darkly. Orthopedics this week. Wayne (PA): RYY Publications; 2009.
71. Joshi D. Extremity market aims for $1billion. Orthopedics this week. Wayne (PA): RRY Publications; 2009.
72. Joshi D. What do the foot and ankle surgeons have to say. Fort Wayne (IN): PeralDiver Technologies; 2008.

Locking Plate Technology and Its Use in Foot and Ankle Surgery

Dekarlos M. Dial, DPM*, Michael Ryan, DPM

KEYWORDS

• Locking plates • Plate design • Fixed-angle plates • Fracture

Over the years, several specialized plates and screws have been developed to manage complex deformities and pathologic bone disorders. Conventional plating systems have traditionally depended on bone quality to achieve and maintain stability. With sufficient cortical bone stiffness and normal bone mineralization, conventional plating systems and bicortical screw fixation can play an important and substantial role toward improving operative outcomes. However, the periarticular anatomy in the foot and ankle may at times prevent use of this particular form of fixation. The result has been the evolution from conventional plating and screw technology to present day fixed-angle devices. Fixed-angle locking plates rely on a different set of mechanical principles. These fixed-angle locking devices minimize compressive forces exerted on the bone by the plate. The plate does not tightly compress against the bone itself to achieve stability.[1] The inherent characteristics of this unique form of fixation aid in periarticular fracture management, achieving skeletal stability in pathologic bone disorders. Combined with the flexibility of traditional plating characteristics, this form of fixation has certainly contributed to the foot and ankle surgeon's operative armamentarium.

In the past, the concept of atraumatic technique, anatomic reduction, rigid internal fixation, and early mobilization as established by the AO group in the late 1950s became the gold standard for surgeons. This approach has been associated with sacrificing the biology of fractures and failing to protect the blood supply of bone in an attempt to precisely reduce fracture fragments.[2,3] Fracture pattern, soft tissue injury, and bone quality critically influence the selection of fixation techniques.[4] The decision to use fixed-angled devices is based on specific anatomic regions, unique fracture patterns, existing implants, and the quality of the bone and soft tissues (**Fig. 1**). Fixed-angle plate osteosynthesis theoretically reduces periosteal trauma and creates a noncompromised biological environment conducive to healing.

Cornerstone Foot and Ankle Specialists, 1814 Westchester Drive, Suite 300, High Point, NC 27262, USA
* Corresponding author.
E-mail address: Dekarlos.Dial@conerstonehealthcare.com

Clin Podiatr Med Surg 28 (2011) 619–631
doi:10.1016/j.cpm.2011.06.003
0891-8422/11/$ – see front matter © 2011 Published by Elsevier Inc.

podiatric.theclinics.com

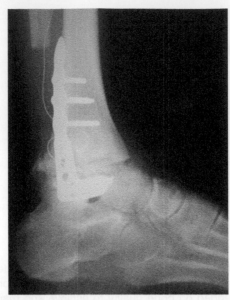

Fig. 1. Radiographs following revision ankle arthrodesis using locking plate construct and implantable bone stimulator.

Locking plates have become widely used, particularly for the treatment of fractures and nonunions.[5–8] This technology undoubtedly assists in both surgical planning and early postoperative rehabilitation. Locking plates provide a higher degree of stability and better protection against primary and secondary losses of reduction while minimizing bone contact.[9–11] Several fixation constructs exist to aid in establishing sufficient and reproducible skeletal stabilization. Precontoured plates also facilitate fixation, placement, and accuracy (**Fig. 2**). This advancement in orthopedic fixation has simplified fracture care and offers a viable alternative when pathologic bone disorders are encountered. In addition, surgical time may be reduced and preoperative planning made easier and less complex.

Most locking plates contain threaded holes into which headless screws can lock. Other designs include special threaded washers that lock the screw to the plate. Such designs provide secure fixation that may provide more stable fixation and allow earlier range of motion (**Fig. 3**). The lower-profile screw heads also reduce soft tissue impingement and hardware irritation.

Even though the initial plating systems were developed for tubular bones, plate design has been modified for improved compatibility with the irregular short bones of the foot. Several companies have developed locking plates for foot and ankle applications that are anatomically shaped, have variable thickness, are made of differing materials, and offer both fixed and angled trajectory. The advances in locking plate fixation may allow for early weight bearing and generate enough stability to negate the motion between the plate and bone.

The objectives of this article are to discuss the history of conventional plating, plate biomechanics, and screw function and provide a better understanding of osseous physiology and biology using locking plates. The authors have researched both peer-reviewed and non–peer-reviewed literature to decipher and share the most pertinent information pertaining to this article.

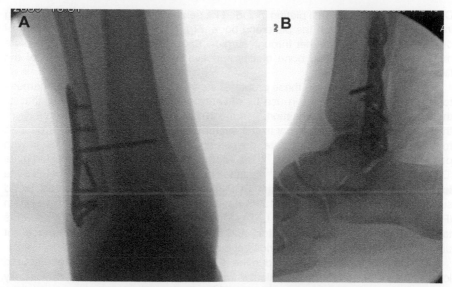

Fig. 2. (*A, B*) Intraoperative fluoroscopic image. Note the lateral precountered plate lateral malleolus.

HISTORY

Plate osteosynthesis began in the late nineteenth century by Hansmann. Later, compression plates were popularized by Danis and the AO group beginning in the late 1950s, introducing concepts and applications for nonlocking plates,[12] which included atraumatic technique, anatomic reduction, rigid internal fixation, and early range of motion. However, traditional plate technology may not be able to produce sufficient torque in cancellous bone in periarticular fractures, comminution, and diseased bone, including osteoporosis.[13] Evolution from nonlocking to fixed-angle devices or locked internal fixation constructs began from these challenges. Traditional plates rely on the friction created between the plate and bone generated by the screw compression. In pathologic bone, the screws in traditional constructs may not generate the compression of bone to plate and so lose overall strength and stability.

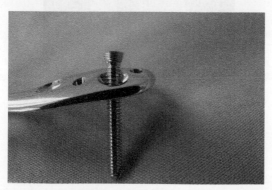

Fig. 3. Locking plate and screw with threads along the undersurface of the screw head to facilitate locking into the plate.

Complications of traditional plating included loosening or toggling of screws resulting in loss of friction between the plate and bone (**Fig. 4**). In addition, the destruction of periosteal blood supply either through surgical dissection or pressure from the plate may lead to compromised bone quality and avascular necrosis in the area of the fixation.[14]

Initial attempts to address these problems included using bone cement to increase torque, but this was limited in use by adverse effects on fracture healing, that is, thermal necrosis and extravasation.[14] In the 1970s and 1980s, the Schuhli nut (Synthes, Paoli, PA, USA) and Zespol fixator systems (Warsaw, Poland) were introduced to allow screws to lock to the plate, preventing toggle of the screw, but issues with periosteal blood supply continued.[15] The Allgower (1971) dynamic compression plate (DCP), modified in 1988 by Perren,[16] included ridges on the inferior surface of the plate to limit overall contact (low-contact DCP [LC-DCP]) and protect periosteal blood supply. Perren and Buchannan (1995) developed the point contact fixator system (PC-Fix; AO; Synthes, Paoli, PA, USA), a unicortical fixation system that prevents toggle with a Morse cone mismatch, and combined this with an undersurface cut out of the LC-DCP to preserve periosteal blood supply.

Refinement of these concepts led to the development of anatomically precontoured locking plates designed for periarticular fractures in the lower extremity, specifically distal femoral and proximal tibial fractures.[17] Precontouring the plate prevented the surgeon from having to bend the plate to match the anatomy. This technique eliminated the deformation of the threaded holes, allowing the screws to lock more accurately. As these plates emerged, the concept of minimally invasive percutaneous osteosynthesis (MIPO) was introduced. With MIPO, the less invasive stabilization system plates were designed to be inserted submuscularly but extraperiosteally. Because they matched the shape of the anatomy, the plates could be slid into place through small incisions. This allowed for preservation of the native biology to the fracture site while reducing possible wound-healing complications.[17]

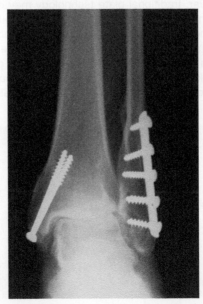

Fig. 4. Traditional plating techniques rely on bone mineralization for achieving fracture stability.

In periarticular fractures, locking compression plates provide improved stability in bone with comminution, and, for many, have replaced the use of blade plate 95° fixed-angle devices.[5] Modern fixed-angle devices now allow locking of a threaded screw head to a threaded plate hole, creating a single beam effect. Locking technology has been applied to all existing plate designs.

The next generation of fixed-angle devices includes variable-angle or polyaxial threaded holes, allowing differing degrees off center, up to 30° with some devices. Other designs include threaded caps to lock the screw to the plate.[18] The threaded holes off center allow screws to capture unique fracture patterns, which, in theory, increases the overall stability in poor bone stock by allowing screws to capture quality bone and apply fixation in multiple planes. Recent clinical data in proximal humerus fractures suggest little difference compared with monoaxial locking technology.[18]

Further refinements have included the development of combination holes, giving the ability of the plate to accommodate both locking and nonlocking screws. This option gives the surgeon the ability to adjust to unique fracture patterns and varying bone quality encountered during surgery.[19]

Locking plates have changed the manner in which complex and osseous conditions are approached. A variety of internal fixation techniques have been used over the years to include wires, staples, screws, plates, and intramedullary devices. Biomechanical studies have proved that some fixation methods offer suboptimal stability, rigidity, and compression (**Fig. 5**). Traditionally, the concept of rigid internal fixation has become the strategic goal of many surgeons. This surgical approach has been linked to sacrificing the biology of the fracture and failure to protect the blood supply of the bone in an effort to anatomically reduce and fix fractures.[2,3,6] The technique of open reduction and internal fixation often requires extensive exposure and visualization and can result in the devitalization of surrounding tissue, infection, wound breakdown, and ankle stiffness.[20] The technique of locked plating was developed in Davos, Switzerland, in the 1990s,[2] and led to a new beginning in plate osteosynthesis.

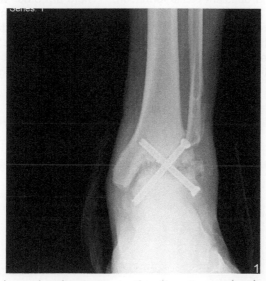

Fig. 5. Noninfected pseudoarthrosis 11 months after attempted arthrodesis using screw fixation.

During its infancy, plates were designed for larger long-bone applications in the upper and lower extremities. In difficult areas, such as those periarticular and in areas of risky anatomy such as the femur,[21] mandible,[22] distal radius,[23] and cervical spine,[24] plates needed to be modified. The plates themselves were too large, and designs to increase the quality and amount of fixation needed to be addressed. From that, small joint systems were developed and have become more used in recent years. The success with the larger earlier devices that were anatomically precontoured led to applying this to smaller locking plates (**Fig. 6**) designed primarily for periarticular fractures of the lower extremities.[25,26] Intuitively, the early rationale in foot and ankle surgery sounds attractive because of the potential to reduce cyclical loading and complications such as hardware failure.

PLATE MECHANICS

With the development of new fixation devices, there has been an increase in biomechanical research and trials. Locking plates have been tested and compared with traditional plates and screws using different constructs.[27,28] Intuitively, the concept of locking plates seems superior to conventional plating, but this hypothesis has not been established in all fracture patterns. In a cadaver study, Redfern and colleagues[27] did not discover any biomechanical advantage over traditional nonlocking plate fixation.

The science of fixed-angle plating systems has emerged as a different category of fixation devices and technological advances. Recently, there has been concern related to the stiffness and rigidity of locking plates in bone healing. The ideal biological environment for comminuted fracture healing relies on bone callus formation.[29,30] In such scenarios, secondary bone healing is stimulated and dependent on controlled interfragmentary motion in the millimeter range.[31] Standard locked plate constructs may be too stiff and lead to asymmetric callus formation along the near cortex, where fracture motion is minimal.[32] In a retrospective series of supracondylar femoral fractures treated with locked plates, the 19% nonunion rate was attributed to attenuated fracture motion and deficient callus formation.[33] There are other variables that can have antagonistic effects on bone healing. Inadequate healing may contribute to increased load bearing of the fixation construct and ultimately hardware fatigue and failure.[34,35] In an alternative strategy to reduce locked plate stiffness without reducing strength, the concept of a far cortical locking plate has been introduced.[36] Far cortical locking screws actually lock into the plate and the far cortex of a long bone to provide

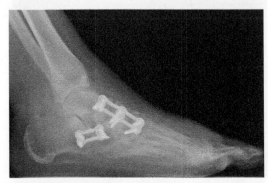

Fig. 6. Radiographs following media lateral foot arthrodesis using anatomically designed locking plates.

parallel interfragmentary motion while maintaining strength and reducing stiffness (**Fig. 7**).[32] In some cases, the periarticular anatomy may impede the use of far cortical locking screws, especially in the foot and ankle regions.

Traditional screw-plate fixation requires bicortical fixation to secure the plate to the bone. The friction generated between the plate and the bone is what gives the stability. However, this construct depends on factors such as bone mineralization and optimal screw purchase to reduce screw toggle. Osteoporotic bone and comminuted bone may prevent generating and maintaining sufficient stability when using conventional plating.

In contrast, the strength of locking plate fixation is the total of all screw-bone interfaces compared with that of a single screw's axial stiffness or pullout resistance as seen in unlocked plates.[13] Locking screws and plates have corresponding thread patterns to facilitate a screw-plate locking connection. Because locked plates do not rely on bone contact for fixation, it is not necessary to pull the bone tightly against the plate. For this reason, locked plates have been called internal-external fixators.[6] Biomechanical testing has provided data favoring locked plate constructs.

BIOMECHANICS OF LOCKING PLATES

Stability determines the amount of strain at the fracture site, and strain determines the type of healing that can occur. Strain is defined as the relative change in fracture gap divided by fracture gap. Primary bone healing occurs when strain is less than 2%, and secondary bone healing occurs when strain is between 2% and 10%. If strain is more than 10%, bone cannot be formed.[9]

One goal of plates is to minimize external forces acting on the bone, including axial, torsional, and 3-point bending. Factors influencing the mechanical stability of a fracture include fracture reduction, number, size and position of screws, plate length, working length, and distance between the plate and bone.[9] The working length of a plate-bone construct is equal to the length of the plate unsupported by bone.[37] For example, bridging plates have long working lengths (**Fig. 8**). As the working length increases, the coronal plane stability decreases. Fixed-angle devices are able to overcome longer working lengths encountered to provide this frontal plane stability. Working length affects axial stiffness and torsional rigidity. Axial compression is influenced by the distance of a screw to the fracture line. Torsional rigidity is determined by the overall number of screws inserted.[38] Increasing the length of a plate increases axial stiffness but has little or no effect on torsion.

Traditional plate mechanics rely on bicortical screws applied through a plate at 1.5 N.[3] Stability results from friction between the undersurface of the plate and bone through bicortical fixation. In locking plates, forces transfer from the bone to the plate exclusively through the screw plate threaded interface. Compression of the plate to

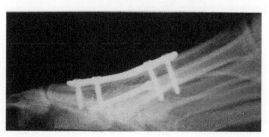

Fig. 7. Far cortical locking technique for first metatarsophalangeal joint arthrodesis.

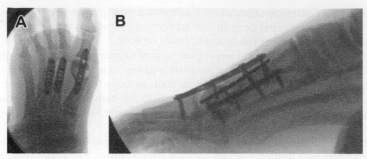

Fig. 8. (*A*) Fluoroscopic image following bridge plating using locking plate for comminuted intra-articular first metatarsal head fracture and adjacent lesser metatarsal fractures. (*B*) Fluoroscopic image of bridge plating using locking plate fixation over the first metatarsophalangeal joint.

the bone is no longer required, allowing for unicortical fixation, although this is not recommended in osteoporotic bone (**Fig. 9**).[39] Unicortical screw fixation provides excess physiologic loads, and the pullout strength of a unicortical locked screw is about 60% the strength of a standard bicortical screw. In situations where excessive torsional loads are expected, bicortical locking screws should be used. Anatomically, metaphyseal bone presents with challenges of decreased bone density and cantilever bending forces, for example, at the medial malleolus. Locking plates accommodate these problems by resisting the moment arm at each individual screw and using unicortical fixation not relying on cancellous bone.

Some principles of external fixation can be applied to these fixed-angle devices. Stability of locking plates is through point fixation, which is analogous to connecting

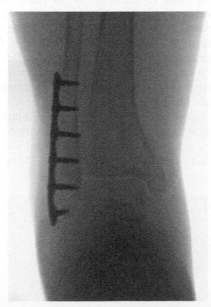

Fig. 9. Intraoperative fluoroscopic image following placement of a unicortical locking plate for a distal lateral malleolar fracture.

bars and pins of an external fixator. Distance from the plate to the bone adversely affects torsional and axial stiffness at greater than 2 mm.[40] Stiffness increases as the plate or bars move closer to the bone, otherwise known as the mechanical axis.[5] Fixed-angle constructs could in theory result in a nonunion generator. Excess stiffness due to the construct in the presence of poor reduction could actually limit the ability of bone to heal. Solutions include increasing the working length of the fracture by skipping holes directly over the fracture to decrease stiffness at the fracture, allowing for secondary or biological healing.[40]

An additional issue with stiffness includes osteoporotic bone and the interface created at the end of the plate. Evidence suggests replacing a locking screw with a nonlocking screw at the last hole to reduce stiffness and risk of periprosthetic fractures.[36]

Optimal screw ratio is equal to the number of screws used divided by the number of available holes. For example a 10-hole plate with 5 screws has a ratio of 0.5. Optimal ratios for bridging plates are 0.4 to 0.5, which equates to 3 to 4 screws above and below the fracture.[41]

DISCUSSION

The evolution of locking plates has been a major advantage in foot and ankle fractures. Even though specific foot and ankle instrumentation lacks substantial medical evidence, the core principles deciphered from larger long-bone literature has allowed for major advancements over the years. These particular fixation methods are being used for the more simplistic conditions to the most advanced and complex deformities one can encounter in foot and ankle surgery.

Gallentine and colleagues[42] published the first series on locking plate fixation for hallux valgus deformities requiring surgical intervention with a proximal first metatarsal chevron osteotomy. The investigators preformed a retrospective review of 20 feet with severe bunion deformities treated with a proximal chevron osteotomy and locking plate fixation. They concluded that the locking plate added stability to the osteotomy and repeatedly held the first ray in good alignment without evidence of transfer lesions or symptomatic hardware. Such reproducibility is desirable in revision bunion surgery or with reduced mineral density.

Achieving adequate fixation while performing tibiotalocalcaneal arthrodesis (TTC) can be a surgical challenge. Various fixation techniques have included screws, traditional plates, blade plate, intramedullary (IM) nails, and external fixation devices. In an attempt to improve stability, reduce technical dilemmas, and attain optimal fixation, several cadaver studies have been performed.[43–45] Chodos and colleagues[43] performed a cadaveric study comparing locking plate versus blade plate strength under dorsiflexion and torsional loading after TTC. In this particular study, the laterally placed periarticular plate group had a higher significant stiffness, higher dorsiflexion, and torsional load to failure and a lower construct deformation than the blade plate group for TTC arthrodesis. This may be attributed to the number of locking screws and the ability to add skeletal stability in multiple planes. A biomechanical investigation demonstrated that a blade plate with a TTC augmentation screw was superior to an IM nail construct that did not include a TTC augmentation screw.[43] The ability to place multiple locking screws in differing planes seems to be of utmost importance from these biomechanical studies.

O'Neil and colleagues[44] performed a cadaver study using 6 matched pairs of fresh frozen cadavers to compare structural rigidity using an IM nail with that using a locking plate, both using a TTC augmentation screw. Even though initial stiffness between the

2 groups was similar in this study, the final stiffness was significantly lower in the IM nail group compared with the locking plate group. The other parameters, including construct deformation, load to failure, and initial stiffness, were statistically insignificant. A major disadvantage of these studies includes the nonphysiologic nature of the cadaver specimens.

Locking plate technology has been one of the major advances in fixation technology over the years. The short and predominantly cancellous bones in the foot increase the difficulty in achieving optimal fixation while avoiding vital soft tissue structures and intra-articular surfaces. Calcaneal fractures may result in severe physical limitations compromising quality of life. Redfern and colleagues[27] used 10 pairs of fresh frozen cadavers to compare the mechanical integrity of locking plate and traditional plate fixation in Sanders type II fractures.[27] In conclusion, the investigators found no biomechanical advantage using locking plates over traditional plate fixation. In a similar mechanical study using a saw bone model, no difference in mean load to failure was found; however, the investigators did report greater rigidity.[28] Regarding early weight bearing, the inherent stability of locking plates may serve to provide greater stability without disrupting fracture stability.[46] The effectiveness of locking plates requires more research to determine the clinical significance.

Saxena and colleagues[47] compared crossed lag screw fixation with a locking plate with a plantar lag screw and concluded that the locking plate and plantar lag screw allowed earlier weight bearing without complication. Another cadaveric study concluded that 2 crossed screws provided stronger fixation in Lapidus arthrodesis than the use of a locking plate without an additional plantar lag screw.[48] A cadaver study using a medial locking plate with adjunct compression screw showed superior stability to the 2 crossed screw construct for a modified Lapidus arthrodesis.[49]

SUMMARY

Locking plate osteosynthesis has evolved over the years with the primary goal to improve surgical outcomes, beginning with traditional plate osteosynthesis and the AO group to present day fixed-angled plates with variable axis. As the technology develops, more research in addition to already existing animal and mechanical models will need to be performed to validate the use of locking plates over traditional compression plating. This research will provide surgeons with a clearer understanding of the indications and limitations of locked plating.

Understanding the mechanics of locked plates is key to understanding the indications and contraindications of this technology. The biology of bone healing is heavily influenced by plate osteosynthesis. Key concepts of stability, strain, and working length allow the surgeon to understand the difference between primary and secondary bone healing. Compression plates provide absolute stability through reducing gap distance and strain. Locked plates function as internal-external fixators, providing stability and strength without compromising periosteal blood supply and functioning as a fixed-angle device. Plate selection should be based on fracture pattern, location, bone, and soft tissue quality.

Impressive union rates have been reported with locking plates; however, the potential for malunion remains a concern.[5] It is important to understand that locking plates are not indicated for every osseous condition requiring fixation. There is also a lack of evidence to support using locking plates in skeletally immature patients and simple fracture patterns. Intraoperatively, it may be difficult to assess bone porosity with the use of locking screws. Once the locking screw engages the locking holes, it can make screw purchase assessment very difficult. Plate bending for locked constructs needs to be done with caution to avoid disrupting the integrity of the hole and threads. One must be careful because this can cross thread the screws, making removal more difficult.

Successful use of locking plates requires careful preoperative planning, consideration of soft tissue dissection principles, and good surgical technique. The frequency of using locked plates is expected to continue to increase with the aging population, periprosthetic fractures, and high-energy trauma. Surgeons must remember that the initial costs of locking plates are substantially more expensive than traditional plating, and the cost/benefit must be determined.

Current advances in locking plate technology have positively influenced use over the years. It is imperative to understand the basic science of conventional plating techniques and plate mechanics before exploring locking plates. After reviewing the literature, the authors found few substantial peer-reviewed studies. In an effort to improve outcomes, the role of locking plates deserves further biomechanical and clinical investigation.

REFERENCES

1. Ronga M, Longo UG, Maffulli N. Minimally invasive locked plating of distal tibia fractures is safe and effective. Clin Orthop Relat Res 2010;468:975–82.
2. Perren SM. Evolution of the internal fixation of long bone fractures: the scientific basis of biological internal fixation. Choosing a new balance between stability and biology. J Bone Joint Surg Br 2002;84:1093–110.
3. Perren SM, Cordey J, Rahn BA, et al. Early temporary porosis of bone induced by internal fixation implants: a reaction to necrosis, not to stress protection? Clin Orthop Relat Res 1988;232:139–51.
4. Bedi A, Lee TT, Karunakar MA. Surgical treatment of nonarticular distal tibia fractures. J Am Acad Orthop Surg 2006;14:406–16.
5. Haidukewych G. Perspectives on modern orthopaedics: innovations in locking plate technology. J Am Acad Orthop Surg 2004;12:205–12.
6. Cantu RV, Koval KJ. The use of locking plates in fracture care. J Am Acad Orthop Surg 2006;14:183–90.
7. Fankhauser F, Boldin C, Schippenger G, et al. A new locking plate for unstable fracture of the proximal humerus. Clin Orthop Relat Res 2005;430:176–81.
8. Ring D, Kline P, Kaczynski J, et al. Locking compression plates for osteoporotic nonunions of the diaphyseal humerus. Clin Orthop Relat Res 2004;425:50–4.
9. Egol K, Kubiak K, Fulkerson E, et al. Biomechanics of locked plates and screws. J Orthop Trauma 2004;18:488–93.
10. Gao H, Zhang CQ, Luo CF, et al. Fractures of the distal tibia treated with polyaxial locking plating. Clin Orthop Relat Res 2009;467:831–7.
11. Kaab MJ, Schmelling FA, Schaser K, et al. Locked internal fixator. Sensitivity of screw/plate stability to the correct insertion angle of the screw. J Orthop Trauma 2004;18:483–7.
12. Bagby GW. Compression bone-plating: historical considerations. J Bone Joint Surg Am 1977;59:625–31.
13. Cordey J, Boregeaud M, Perren SM. Force transfer between the plate and the bone: relative importance of the bending stiffness of the screws friction between plate and bone. Injury 2000;31(Suppl 3):C21–8.
14. Kubiak E, Fulkerson E, Strauss E, et al. The evolution of locked plates. J Bone Joint Surg Am 2006;88:189–200.
15. Ramotowski W, Granowski R. Zespol: an original method of stable osteosynthesis. Clin Orthop 1991;272:67–75.

16. Perren SM. Point contact fixator: part I. Scientific background, design and application. Injury 1995;22(S1):1–10.
17. Schandelmaier P. LISS osteosynthesis for distal fractures of the femur. Trauma und Berufskrankheit 1999;1:392–7.
18. Ockert B, Braunstein V, Kirchoff C, et al. Monoaxial versus polyaxial screw insertion in angular stable plate fixation of proximal humerus fractures: radiographic analysis of a prospective randomized study. J Trauma 2010;69:1545–51.
19. Frigg R. Development of the locking compression plate. Injury 2003;34:S-B6–10.
20. Teeney SM, Wiss DA. Open reduction and internal fixation of tibial plafond fractures. Clin Orthop Relat Res 1993;292:108–17.
21. Kregor PJ, Hughes JL, Cole PA. Distal femoral fracture fixation utilizing the Less Invasive Stabilization System (L.I.S.S.): the technique and early results. Injury 2001;32(Suppl 3):SC32–47.
22. Drobertz H, Kutscha-Lissberg E. Osteosynthesis of distal radius fractures with a volar locking screw plate system. Int Orthop 2003;27:1–6.
23. Schutz M, Muller M, Krettek C, et al. Minimally invasive fracture stabilization of distal femoral fractures with the LISS: a prospective multicenter study: results of a clinical study with special emphasis on difficult cases. Injury 2001;32(Suppl 3): SC48–54.
24. Spivak JM, Chen D, Kummer FJ. The effect of locking fixation screws on the stability of anterior cervical plating. Spine 1999;24:334–8.
25. Haidukewych GL. Innovations in locking plate technology. J Am Acad Orthop Surg 2004;12:205–12.
26. Korner J, Lill H, Muller LP, et al. The LCP—concept in the operative treatment of distal humerus fractures-biological, biomechanical and surgical aspects. Injury 2003;34(Suppl 2):B20–30.
27. Redfern DJ, Oliveira ML, Campbell JT, et al. A biomechanical comparison of locking plates and nonlocking plates for the fixation of calcaneal fractures. Foot Ankle Int 2006;27:196–201.
28. Richter M, Gosling T, Zech S, et al. A comparison of plates with and without locking screws in a calcaneal fracture model. Foot Ankle Int 2005;26:309–19.
29. Hente R, Fuchtmeier B, Schlegel U, et al. The influence of cyclic compression and distraction on the healing of experimental tibial fractures. J Orthop Res 2004;22:709–15.
30. Claes LE, Heigele CA, Neidlinger-Wilke C, et al. Effects of mechanical factors on the fracture healing process. Clin Orthop Relat Res 1998;355(Suppl):S132–47.
31. Rahn BA, Gallinaro P, Baltensperger A, et al. Primary bone healing. An experimental study in the rabbit. J Bone Joint Surg Am 1971;53:783–6.
32. Bottlang M, Lesser M, Koerber K, et al. Far cortical locking plates can improve healing of fractures stabilized with locking plates. J Bone Joint Surg Am 2010;92: 1652–60.
33. Lujan TJ, Henderson CE, Madey SM, et al. Locked plating of distal femur fractures leads to inconsistent and asymmetric callus formation. J Orthop Trauma 2010;24:156–62.
34. Kregor PJ, Stannard JA, Zlowodzki M, et al. Treatment of distal femur fractures using the less invasive stabilization system: surgical experience and early clinical results in 103 fractures. J Orthop Trauma 2004;18:509–20.
35. Fankhauser F, Gruber G, Schippinger G, et al. Minimal invasive treatment of the LISS (Less Invasive Stabilization System): a prospective study of 30 fractures with a follow up of 20 months. Acta Orthop Scand 2004;75:55–60.

36. Bottlang M, Doornink J, Fitzpatrick DC, et al. Far cortical locking can reduce stiffness of locked plating constructs while retaining construct strength. J Bone Joint Surg Am 2009;91:1985.
37. Mast J, Jakob R, Ganz R. Planning and reduction technique in fracture surgery. Berlin: Springer-Verlag; 1989.
38. Stoffel K, Dieter U, Stachowiak G, et al. Biomechanical testing of the LCP—how can stability in locked internal fixators be controlled? Injury 2003;34(Suppl 2): B11-9.
39. Talbot M, Zdero R, Garneau D, et al. Fixation of long bone segmental defects: a biomechanical study. Injury 2008;39:181-6.
40. Ahmad M, Nanda R, Bajwa AS, et al. Biomechanical testing of the locking compression plate: when does the distance between bone and implant significantly reduce construct stability? Injury 2007;38:358-64.
41. Gautier E, Sommer C. Guidelines for the clinical application of the LCP. Injury 2003;34(Suppl 2):B63-76.
42. Gallentine JW, DeOrio JK, DeOrio MJ. Bunion surgery using locking-plate fixation of proximal chevron osteotomies. Foot Ankle Int 2007;28:361-8.
43. Chodos MD, Brent PG, Schon LC, et al. Blade plate compared with locking plate for tibiotalocalcaneal arthrodesis: a cadaver study. Foot Ankle Int 2008;29: 219-24.
44. O'Neil PJ, Logel KJ, Parks BG, et al. Rigidity comparison of locking plate intramedullary fixation for tibiotalocalcaneal arthrodesis. Foot Ankle Int 2008;29:581-6.
45. Chiodo CP, Acevedo JI, Sammarco VJ, et al. Intramedullary fixation compared with blade-plate- and screw fixation for tibiotalocalcaneal arthrodesis: a biomechanical investigation. J Bone Joint Surg Am 2003;85:2425-8.
46. Hyer CF, Atway S, Berlet GC, et al. Early weight bearing of calcaneal fractures fixated with locked plates: a radiographic review. Foot Ankle Spec 2010;3:320-3.
47. Saxena A, Nguyen A, Nelsen E. Lapidus bunionectomy: early evaluation of crossed lag screws versus locking plate with plantar lag screw. J Foot Ankle Surg 2009;48:170-9.
48. Cohen DA, Parks BG, Schon LC. Screw fixation compared to H-locking fixation for first metatarsal cuneiform joint arthrodesis: a biomechanical study. Foot Ankle Int 2005;26:984-9.
49. Klos K, Gueroguiev B, Muckley T, et al. Stability of medial locking plate and a compression screw versus two crossed screws for Lapidus arthrodesis. Foot Ankle Int 2010;31:158-63.

Advances in Intramedullary Nail Fixation in Foot and Ankle Surgery

Jason B. Woods, DPM*, Patrick R. Burns, DPM

KEYWORDS

- Tibiotalocalcaneal • Intramedullary nail • Foot • Ankle
- Arthrodesis

Fracture care of long bones in both upper and lower extremities has employed intramedullary (IM) nail fixation for many years. Its use in reconstructive foot and ankle surgery has a shorter history and has been slower to develop. However, in the past 2 decades it has been steadily gaining popularity.

The first description of IM fixation for ankle arthrodesis was by Lexer[1] in 1906. His technique, termed Bolzungs arthrodese, consisted of placing boiled corpse bone through a hole in the calcaneus, talus, and tibia. Albee[2] modified this technique, harvesting an autogenous vertical spike of fibula and inserting this through the calcaneus, talus, and tibia, in 1915.

Adams[3] is credited with the first published results of ankle arthrodesis using a retrograde metallic nail. The author used a 3-flanged trifin nail for fixation. Although this construct did not have any interlocking screws, his report of 30 patients noted only 2 failures. In 1950, Leikkonen[4] followed suit using a metal spike, which was removed after 10 days. Bingold[5] inserted fibular graft after using a cannulated drill over a guidewire placed through the calcaneus, talus, and tibia. In 1967, Küntscher[6] described the use of an unlocked retrograde conical-shaped nail for tibiotalocalcaneal arthrodesis.

In the early 1990s, IM nails with interlocking screws became available for hindfoot arthrodesis. Stone and Helal[7] reported achieving arthrodesis in 19 of 20 patients, with weight bearing allowed at 2 weeks after surgery.

The use of IM nail fixation in foot and ankle surgery is generally reserved for lower-extremity salvage procedures, where gross instability, severe misalignment, and end-stage arthrosis are common. Situations that may require IM nail fixation include

University of Pittsburgh Medical Center, Comprehensive Foot and Ankle Center, Roesch-Taylor Medical Building, 2100 Jane Street, Suite 7100 North, Pittsburgh, PA 15203, USA
* Corresponding author. 1400 Locust Street, Pittsburgh, PA 15219.
E-mail address: woodsJb@upmc.edu

Clin Podiatr Med Surg 28 (2011) 633–648
doi:10.1016/j.cpm.2011.06.004
0891-8422/11/$ – see front matter © 2011 Elsevier Inc. All rights reserved.

Charcot neuroarthropathy, avascular necrosis of the talus, failed total ankle arthroplasty, previous failed attempts at hindfoot or ankle arthrodesis procedures, or severe posttraumatic arthritis.[8] These situations are frequently complicated by diabetes mellitus, peripheral neuropathy, peripheral arterial disease, neuromuscular disorders, and rheumatologic arthridities.

COMPLICATIONS

Complications encountered with tibiotalocalcaneal (TTC) arthrodesis using IM nails include nonunion, malunion, delayed union, infection, periprosthetic fracture (**Fig. 1**), hardware failure (**Fig. 2**), lateral plantar nerve injury, and wound healing difficulties. In general, the overall complication rates of hindfoot arthrodesis for complex deformities are high, experienced in 15% to 80% according to published reports.[9–14]

Because of the prevalence of complex foot and ankle deformities in diabetic neuropathic patients, TTC arthrodesis procedures may be associated with an increased overall complication rate compared with other elective orthopaedic procedures. Wukich and colleagues[15] found that diabetic patients were 5 times more likely to develop an infection requiring hospitalization, with complicated diabetics having an increased infection rate by a factor of 10 compared with nondiabetics. Furthermore, when studying diabetic patients who suffered an ankle fracture, the same author[16] found that patients with complicated diabetes have a 3.8 times greater risk of overall complications, 3.4 times greater risk of noninfectious complications, and 5 times greater risk of requiring further surgery compared with patients with uncomplicated diabetes. The increased risk of complications must be carefully considered by the surgeon, and thoroughly discussed with the patient, before undertaking complex hindfoot arthrodesis within this patient population.

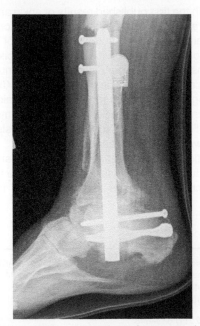

Fig. 1. A periprosthetic fracture at the proximal tip of a retrograde femoral nail used for TTC arthrodesis in a diabetic neuropathic patient.

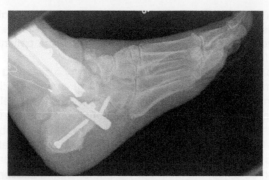

Fig. 2. Hardware failure at distal aspect of IM nail in a diabetic neuropathic patient following attempted TTC arthrodesis. The patient only complained of a squeaking sound during ambulation, as the broken ends of the nail rubbed.

TECHNICAL CONSIDERATIONS

The technical aspects of inserting an IM nail for TTC arthrodesis can be demanding. Most devices used today allow for a cannulated insertion technique using a guidewire. In normal anatomy, the calcaneus is located laterally and inferior to the tibia, requiring either medialization of the hindfoot or the use of a valgus-angulated nail for proper placement. However, many deformities requiring IM fixation do not have normal anatomy and proper preoperative and intraoperative planning is advised.

Approaches for joint preparation vary widely based on the deformity that exists. Each approach has its advantages and disadvantages. When choosing an approach, the presence and location of ulcerations, previous surgical scars, or skin grafts and/or flaps must be considered because these may affect incision options for the surgeon. Deformities must also be considered that may need to be corrected with osteotomies.

Perhaps the most popular approach is the transfibular approach. A lateral incision is made over the fibula and extending along the lateral foot just superior to the course of the peroneal tendons. A fibular osteotomy is required to gain access to the joint, and is performed approximately 5 cm above the ankle mortise. The fibula can then be completely removed from the field and placed in normal saline on the back table for later use as graft. This technique allows great exposure to the ankle and subtalar joint. All cartilage is then removed from the talar dome and tibia followed by the posterior articular facets of the subtalar joint. Joint surfaces are then be "fish-scaled" with an osteotome and drilled with a kirschner wire to break through the subchondral plate to prepare for arthrodesis. Care must be taken to ensure that the joint is prepared properly, because an uneven preparation can result in an iatrogenic varus or valgus deformity. It is the senior author's experience that special attention must be paid to avoid removing too much cartilage and subchondral bone laterally, because this is the aspect of the joint that is most visible when using the transfibular approach. It is our recommendation to start denuding at the most medial aspect of the joint possible, and work laterally when preparing the joint surfaces.

Once the joints are prepared, the previously excised fibula can then serve as a source of autogenous bone graft. It can be split longitudinally, harvesting the medial one-third of the fibula as autogenous graft. If needed, this material can be mixed with commercially available demineralized bone matrix to increase to an appropriate volume, which is then introduced into the ankle and subtalar joints. In many cases, the remaining two-thirds of the fibula is placed back onto the lateral surface of the ankle to serve as a biologic onlay graft. This technique provides a biologic plate to the arthrodesis site, as well as increasing the possibility that the ankle fusion could be taken down in favor of a total ankle replacement should the patient not tolerate an arthrodesis in the future.

At this point, the foot and ankle is placed in position for fusion. Leg holding devices, such as bone foam, stacked sterile towels, or modified external fixation components, can aid the surgeon with positioning. The foot is placed 90 degrees in relation to the distal leg, with approximately 10 to 15 degrees of foot external rotation in the transverse plane, with care to make the operative limb symmetric to the contralateral limb. The second toe is aligned with the tibial crest. The calcaneus should be in approximately 5 degrees of valgus. The talus is translated posteriorly within the ankle mortise approximately 5 mm.

With the position obtained, the ideal entry point for the IM fixation must be determined. Once again, the deformity being treated must be carefully considered when choosing a starting point. In most cases, the calcaneus is located lateral to the talus, requiring some degree of medialization of the calcaneus and/or the use of a valgus-oriented IM nail. Fluoroscopy is mandatory and allows visualization of the initial guide-wire placement. Using axial calcaneal, lateral, and anteroposterior (AP) ankle views, proper placement can be ensured. The initial guide pin should bisect the calcaneus on the axial view. On the lateral view, the lateral process of the talus will be superimposed over the guide wire. The guide wire should appear to be bisecting the width of lateral process of the talus for optimal positioning. The guide wire is then advanced into the distal tibia. An AP view of the ankle confirms proper placement through the middle of the talus, and the wire should be centered within the distal tibia.

A reproducible description for obtaining a starting point was described by Belczyk and colleagues.[17] A metallic rod or guidewire can be used to determine the longitudinal location bisecting the lateral process of the talus and distal tibia on lateral C-arm view (**Fig. 3**). Once the position is ideal, a skin marker is used to mark the location of the rod on the lateral aspect of the ankle. This line is then continued plantarly from lateral to medial across the calcaneus. Next, the axial location of the entry point is determined in a similar way. An axial calcaneal C-arm image is obtained with the threaded rod bisecting the hindfoot on the plantar aspect of the calcaneus. This location is then traced with the skin marker. The ideal entry point is located where the 2 lines intersect (**Fig. 4**).

Once the guidewire is placed, the first cannulated drill is used to break into the distal tibia. If the drill being used has both a reaming and drilling setting, ensure that the device is set to drill. The drill is advanced through the calcaneus, talus, and into the tibia until just the distal subchondral plate is violated. Once the canal is open, the short guide pin is exchanged for a ball-tipped guide wire for the reaming process.

Cannulated reamers are used to slowly increase the diameter of the medullary canal. Because reaming generates a large amount of heat, it is advised that the tourniquet is deflated for this portion of the procedure. This allows for blood to serve as a coolant. In addition, dropping the tourniquet during reaming may decrease the likelihood of accumulation of fat emboli with subsequent release when the tourniquet is discontinued at the end of the case, in favor of the gradual release of smaller emboli during the reaming process. Continue reaming until the canal has been reamed to 1.5 mm greater than the desired nail (eg, for a nail with a diameter of 10 mm, ream to 11.5 mm). Take care during this process because you may still affect change in position. If the position is not secured, the foot may fall into plantarflexion or other deformities while reaming and affect the end product.

At this point, the nail length and diameter are chosen. The nail is then positioned on the insertion jig. It is important to be familiar with this step. Each company is unique,

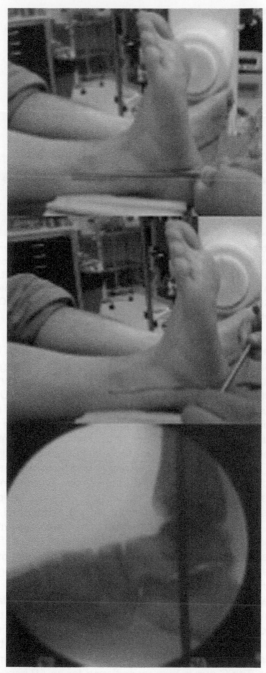

Fig. 3. Using C-arm, a line is made on the lateral aspect of the ankle corresponding to bisection of the distal tibia and the lateral process of the talus. The line is then extended across the plantar calcaneus. (*From* Belczyk RJ, Sung W, Wukich DK. Technical tip: a simple method for proper placement of an intramedullary nail entry point for tibiotalocalcaneal or tibiocalcaneal Arthrodesis. Foot Ankle Online J 2008;1(9):6; with permission.)

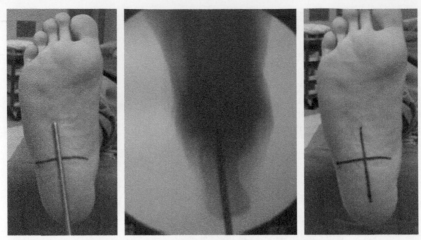

Fig. 4. A metallic object is then placed along the plantar calcaneus. C-arm is used to ensure bisection of the hindfoot. A line is then traced on the skin. Intersection of these 2 lines represents the ideal entry point for guidewire placement. (*From* Belczyk RJ, Sung W, Wukich DK. Technical tip: a simple method for proper placement of an intramedullary nail entry point for tibiotalocalcaneal or tibiocalcaneal Arthrodesis. Foot Ankle Online J 2008;1(9): 6, 7; with permission.)

with different screw locations and orientations. It is imperative to have the correct alignment of the nail on the jig or the locking screws may not engage the nail.

Now that the canal is reamed to the appropriate diameter and the nail prepared, the cannulated jig is used to insert the nail over the ball-tip guidewire. Using C-arm visualization, a mallet is used to advance the nail until it is flush or slightly recessed into the calcaneus depending on patient anatomy and nail design. From this point, the procedure may differ based on the specifications of the nail being implanted.

For most IM devices, attention is then directed to the interlocking screws. Most designs start with fixation distally. The calcaneus and possibly talus are fixed using the jig for guidance. If available, the construct may now be compressed before the interlocking tibial screws are placed for final fixation. For most devices, the proximal screws can be inserted using the company jig. At the shorter nail lengths used for TTC applications, the jig remains accurate. For longer nails, a jig may not hold true and the proximal locking screws must be placed freehand.

For freehand placement of screws in the tibia, the importance of proper use of fluoroscopy cannot be overstated. The C-arm must be completely orthogonal to the operative extremity. Using a lateral image, the medial-to-lateral holes in the proximal portion of the rod are visualized. The holes must be completely circular, which ensures that there is no unwanted oblique angulation. The drill is placed on the surface of the skin and visualized under the C-arm. Once a small skin incision is made, the senior author's preferred technique is to put the drill tip on the bone at the most anterior aspect of the interlocking screw hole. Once there, the drill is dropped to a position parallel to the floor. The C-arm is then repositioned for an AP image of the proximal tibia and the position of the drill in relation to the hole is once again verified. The medial cortex of the tibia is penetrated. When the drill tip is within the medullary canal and the hole in the rod, the drill bit is detached from the drill and the bit is advanced using a mallet to avoid unnecessary heat generation. This method also allows the drill bit to take the path of least resistance, accommodating for minor errors in position.

The bit is advanced through the nail to the other cortex. Once the bit has traversed the tibia, the drill is reattached and a hole in the lateral cortex of the tibia is drilled. The drill is then removed and the proximal screw measured and inserted.

For some IM nails, an oblong dynamization hole is present in the proximal aspect. If so desired, care is taken to insert the screw into the most proximal aspect of this hole to allow the nail to be dynamized later if necessary. This dynamization hole allows the nail to slide proximally, allowing dynamic compression of the arthrodesis site with weightbearing, thus potentially stimulating bone healing. The screw that remains in this hole allows movement in an axial direction but still limits rotation of the nail, which would be detrimental (this is discussed later).

VALGUS-ORIENTED NAILS

One of the first questions when planning for a TTC arthrodesis is whether a straight or curved nail should be used.[18] Difficulties encountered when using IM nails not designed specifically for hindfoot anatomy have been reported.[18–20] In recent years, more hindfoot-specific designs have been made available, increasing the interest in comparing the use of straight versus curved nails. Inherently, placing an IM nail retrograde through the plantar surface of the foot places neurovascular and myotendinous structures at significant risk for damage.[21,22] The use of a valgus nail may be helpful in avoiding some of the more vital structures in this region and more closely reproduces the normal anatomy.

A cadaveric study comparing a straight hindfoot nail (Biomet Ankle Arthrodesis Nail, Biomet, Berlin, Germany) with a hindfoot-specific–designed nail with a 5-degree valgus bend (Ankle Arthrodesis Nail, Stryker, Schoenkirchen, Germany) supports the use of a valgus-curved nail to avoid destruction of important anatomic structures.[18] The entry point on the plantar surface of the heel was significantly closer to the medial plantar artery, the lateral plantar nerve, and the flexor hallucis longus tendon when using the straight nail compared with the curved nail, implying that damage could be inflicted more frequently with a straight nail. The damage to the peroneus brevis caused by insertion of the lateral-to-medial interlocking screw of the straight nail was statistically significant compared with the valgus nail. This cadaveric study suggests that less iatrogenic damage is caused with the use of a 5-degree valgus hindfoot nail.

In a recent study, Budnar and colleagues[23] report on their series of TTC arthrodesis procedures on 45 patients using a short valgus-oriented hindfoot nail (DePuy Versa-Nail) The investigators report clinical and radiographic union in 40/45 patients (89%). The mean postoperative American Orthopaedic Foot and Ankle Society (AOFAS) score was 69, with a mean improvement of 37 points compared with preoperative scores. When excluding the 5 nonunions, these values improved to 76 and 42 respectively. The investigators report only 1 incident of mild plantar nerve irritation, which did not require further surgery. The investigators credit the more laterally located entry point used for the valgus nail for the limited number of iatrogenic plantar injuries.

Not all patients have the normal or required anatomy for the valgus nail designs. In certain disorders, such as Charcot neuroarthropathy, the talus may be severely deformed or even absent. In these types of cases, a straight nail may be more beneficial. There may not be the need to medialize the distal segment, or, if the talus is absent, the missing height may change the position of the valgus bend. Without the proper height, the bend occurs within the tibia and may interfere with overall position (**Fig. 5**).

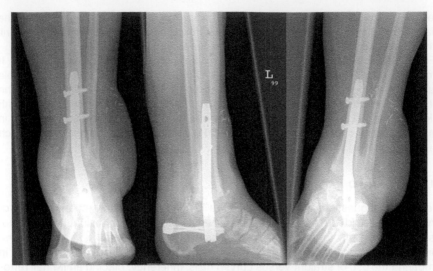

Fig. 5. Radiographs depicting a hindfoot-specific valgus-oriented IM nail inserted after failed total ankle arthroplasty. Note the loss of height of the talus, resulting in the valgus bend of the IM nail being too proximal within the distal tibia.

SCREW ORIENTATION

Most first-generation nails were designed with coronal interlocking screws that could only be placed perpendicular to the IM nail. With the production of second-generation nails, screws can now be placed in different orientations and angulations than previously were available.

The most obvious change to screw orientation has been the adoption of a posterior-to-anterior position of the calcaneal interlocking screws (**Fig. 6**). Mann and colleagues[24] were the first to compare the use of posterior-to-anterior screw placement within the calcaneus with the more traditional lateral-to-medial orientation. This cadaveric study showed that the posterior-to-anterior screws resulted in 40% more stiffness. These findings were confirmed by Means and colleagues,[25] who found that calcaneal screws placed posterior to anterior, rather than lateral to medial, resulted in higher values for fatigue endurance load to failure, higher final stiffness, and lower plastic deformation.

As designs continue to evolve, oblique screw holes have become available. Oblique holes allow the surgeon to achieve fixation through multiple bones with 1 interlocking screw (**Fig. 7**). For example, the Trigen Hindfoot Fusion Nail (Smith and Nephew) has an obliquely oriented distal calcaneal screw that allows posterior-to-anterior fixation starting within the calcaneus and crossing the subtalar joint into the talus. The 55-degree angle of this hole in relation to the IM nail provides additional fixation options. With the use of a longer screw, fixation across the talonavicular joint in addition to the subtalar joint may be accomplished.

DYNAMIZATION

Most second-generation hindfoot nails have oblong holes that can be used for dynamization (**Fig. 8**). Dynamization is defined as altering the nail construct to allow for some motion in the form of compression when the limb is loaded, Dynamization is performed

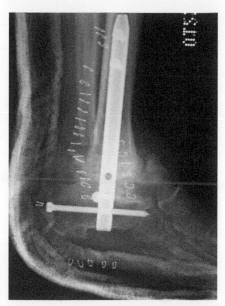

Fig. 6. Posterior-to-anterior screw placement distally within the calcaneus.

with the hope that this movement will stimulate further healing of the arthrodesis site. By removing neighboring static screws but leaving the screw in the oblong hole intact, controlled micromotion in permitted axially, but rotation is not.

In foot and ankle applications, IM rods are dynamized by removing proximal screws. The distal screws are left in place, preventing distal migration of the rod through the

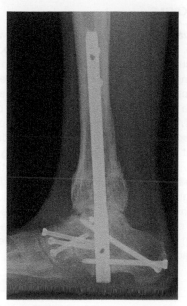

Fig. 7. IM nail with angulated screw from plantar-posterior calcaneus passing obliquely into talar body.

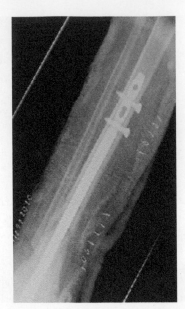

Fig. 8. An oblong dynamization hole in proximal aspect of an IM nail.

plantar aspect of the heel, where it would become prominent. With the proximal static screw removed, the rod instead migrates within the tibial canal proximally.

Oblong holes can also be used within internal compression devices within the distal interlocking screw holes. Internal compression devices push the screw located in the oblong hole toward the arthrodesis site, thereby causing compression.

FIXED-ANGLE LOCKING SCREWS

Screws holes are now available with fixed-angle, also known as angle-stable, technology. This technology is accomplished by the interlocking screw hole being threaded, or the screw cutting threads within the hole with the IM nail on insertion. This results in a fixed-angle relationship between the interlocking screws and IM nail (**Fig. 9**). This construct may allow for increased rigidity and stability.

The use of angle-stable screws was studied in synthetic bone models and human cadaveric specimens by Mückley and colleagues.[26] The investigators studied Stryker T2 nails with fixed-angle screws and fixed-angle screws under compression to a statically locked nail (Biomet Ankle Arthrodesis Nail, Germany). Nails with fixed-angle screws outperformed the non–fixed-angle constructs in initial stability and following cyclical loading testing in both synthetic and cadaveric models. The non–fixed-angle construct showed 5 fatigue failures in 8 trials of cyclical loading compared with 1 failure of 8 trials for both the noncompressed and compressed fixed-angle constructs. Kasper and colleagues[27] showed similar results using angle-stable constructs for IM fixation of sheep tibiae. In this study, the use of angle-stable fixation increased interfragmentary rigidity and accelerated overall healing rates.

SPIRAL BLADE SCREWS

Spiral blade screws have been used in the treatment of hip fractures for many years. This device increases the surface area of the bone-to-implant interface compared with

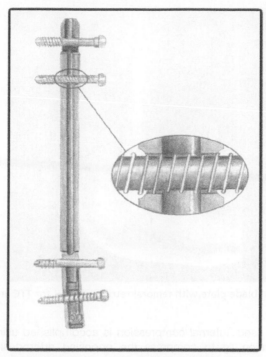

Fig. 9. Typical IM nail fixed-angle screw mechanism proximally and internal compression mechanism distally. (*Based on the work of* Muckley T, Hoffmeier K, Klos K, et al. Angle-stable and compressed angle-stable locking for tibiotalocalcaneal arthrodesis with retrograde intramedullary nails. Biomechanical evaluation. J Bone Joint Surg Am 2008;90(3):621; with permission.)

a traditional screw. Spiral blades may be placed from the posterior aspect of the calcaneus, through a fixed-angle hole within the IM nail in certain models. This feature can be useful when dealing with osteopenic bone, because the increased surface area allows a more rigid fixation construct (**Fig. 10**). Being a largely cancellous bone, the use of a spiral blade within the calcaneus may be advantageous.

In a cadaveric study, Klos and colleagues[28] found that the use of a fixed-angle posterior-to-anterior spiral blade and conventional fixed-angle screw used in the calcaneus was superior to 2 conventional fixed-angle screws in the calcaneus with the Synthes Hindfoot Arthrodesis Expert Nailing System. The addition of the spiral blade resulted in a significantly more rigid construct with dorsiflexion/plantarflexion loading. In addition, correlation with bone mineral density analysis of the cadaveric specimens suggests that the spiral blade may be especially useful for patients with poor bone stock.[28]

ACHIEVEMENT OF COMPRESSION

Achieving stiffness with any TTC arthrodesis construct is desirable. Multiple studies suggest that IM nails may provide more stiffness than screw constructs.[29,30] Achieving compression across the arthrodesis site is crucial to biomechanical stability and initial construct stiffness when performing TTC fusion,[31,32] as shown in cadaveric studies.

Compression across the arthrodesis site can be accomplished using either internally derived compression or externally derived compression, depending on the IM

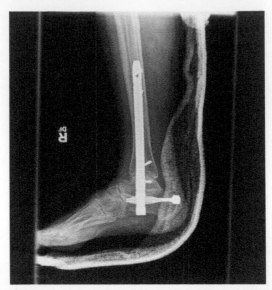

Fig. 10. Use of spiral blade plate with femoral retrograde nail for TTC arthrodesis.

nail system being used. Internal compression is accomplished using a mechanism within the application jig to compress the opposing arthrodesis surfaces (see **Fig. 9**), whereas external compression requires placement of separate pins within the tibia to generate compressive forces (**Fig. 11**). Therefore, external compression mechanisms are more invasive. Both the DePuy VersaNail and Integra Panta Nail use external compression devices.

Muckley[26] found that constructs with compressed fixed-angle IM nails outperformed noncompressed fixed-angle constructs against internal/external rotational forces in synthetic bone models, but no statistically significant difference was detected in cadaveric models. Both compressed and noncompressed IM nails showed failure in 1 out of 8 models, with failure occurring at the posterior-to-anterior calcaneal screw for each model. The investigators postulate that there was no benefit shown in the cadaveric models as a result of hardware loosening because of cancellous bone as well as impaction of the opposing joint surfaces that occurs with

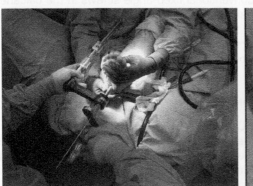
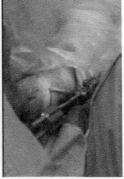

Fig. 11. Jig with external compression device using tibial pins (VersaNail, DePuy).

the generation of compression. In addition, the talar screw showed loosening following cyclical loading in 1 case of the compressed fixed-angle model. The force applied to the talar screw when the internal compression screw is applied may serve as a cause of potential screw loosening within the talus.

Yakacki and coworkers[33] compared the achievement and maintenance of compression of IM nail fixation (New Deal/Integra Panta Nail and DePuy Versa Nail) with external ring fixators in cadaveric specimens and synthetic bone models. Both IM nails tested feature external tibial pins that may be used to generate compressive forces during implantation. The investigators found that the Panta Nail device construct was capable of generating high levels of compressive forces during implantation. The VersaNail generated approximately 20% of the force generated by the Panta Nail; however, both IM nail constructs lost 90% of the load generated during implantation once the external implantation devices were removed. In contrast, the external ring fixator models were able to generate high levels of compression, with maintenance of 50% of the load after simulated bone resorption occurred. External fixation models caused 4 mm of simulated bone resorption, compared with less than 1 mm of resorption with the IM nail constructs. The investigators conclude that IM nails are unable to provide sustained compression once bone resorption occurs. The need for further investigation of the biologic response to bone resorption and compression across an arthrodesis site was also highlighted.

Niinimaki and colleagues[14] used an IM nail with nail-mounted external compression device (Biomet, Warsaw, IN, USA) while performing TTC arthrodesis in 34 patients. The investigators experienced an overall union rate of 76% at a mean of 16 weeks. Of their 4 reported postoperative infections, 2 necessitated implant removal. Three patients required revision of the arthrodesis because of pain.

COMPARISON OF IM NAILS WITH OTHER FORMS OF FIXATION

Numerous biomechanical studies comparing IM nail fixation with other forms of TTC arthrodesis fixation have been performed with varying results. This variability in results can most likely be attributed to the use of different IM nails with a large variance in technological features.

Berend[29] found that IM nails with lateral-to-medial distal screws outperformed crossed screws in biomechanical stiffness. Chiodo[34] found that a humeral blade plate with an additional 6.5-mm cancellous screw had greater stiffness compared with a supracondylar IM rod (DePuy) used for TTC arthrodesis. The use of an augmentation screw within the blade plate design initiated interest in adding an augmentation screw to IM nail constructs. O'Neil and colleagues[35] investigated IM nail fixation augmented with an additional screw placed from the plantar-posterior aspect of the calcaneus to the anteromedial aspect of the distal tibia versus IM nail fixation alone. The investigators found significantly higher initial and final stiffness with the use of an extra augmentation screw. When bone mineral density of the cadaveric specimens was investigated, a negative correlation was found between decreased bone mineral density and fixation performance in those without an augmentation screw. The investigators conclude that an augmentation screw may be of particular benefit with osteoporotic patients. In a subsequent study, O'Neil and colleagues[36] investigated locking plates compared with IM nails in a cadaveric study. The final stiffness values of a locking plate with augmentation screw construct was shown to be superior to that of an IM nail (Biomet) with augmentation screw construct; however, no difference in initial stiffness was observed, with no construct failures experienced in either group.

A few studies have compared the biomechanical properties of IM nails with blade plate fixation in TTC arthrodesis procedures. Lee and colleagues[37] used cadaveric models to compare the biomechanical fatigue endurance and load to failure of IM nail construct versus blade plate with 6.5-mm cancellous compression screw construct for tibiocalcaneal arthrodesis. The investigators conclude that the IM nail construct provided greater stiffness and was biomechanically superior to the blade-plate-and-screw construct. Recently, Froelich and colleagues[38] found no statistically significant difference between IM nail fixation and a lateral blade-plate-and-screw construct in a cadaveric biomechanical study. Similar results were reported by Alfahd and colleagues,[39] who found a statistically significant decrease in internal rotation strength when comparing the lateral blade plate with the IM nail (ReVision IM Nail, Smith and Nephew). Both studies show a trend toward improved performance of the IM nail constructs in specimens with decreased bone mineral density.

External fixation constructs have also been compared with IM nail constructs. Santangelo and coworkers[40] compared IM nail fixation (VersaNail, DePuy Orthopaedics, Warsaw, IN, USA) with external circular ring fixation using matched pairs of cadaveric specimens for TTC arthrodesis. No difference was found between the 2 fixation methods in bending stiffness, but external fixation outperformed the IM nail in resisting torsional stress in both internal and external rotation. The investigators concluded that, although both constructs provide satisfactory fixation, the external ring fixator provides a stiffer construct with a statistically significant superior performance against rotational forces. This study is supported by the work of Fragomen and colleagues,[41] who found no significant difference between external fixation and IM nailing in a similarly designed biomechanical cadaveric experiment.

SUMMARY

Hindfoot arthrodesis in the treatment of complex foot and ankle deformities are extremely challenging cases. Technological advances in IM nail fixation have improved the biomechanical properties of available fixation constructs in recent years. Although advances may help to improve clinical results, small sample sizes and the low-level evidence of study designs limit the evaluation of the benefits of these advances in clinical outcomes.

ACKNOWLEDGMENTS

The authors would like to thank Kristy Hartman for producing illustrations within the article.

REFERENCES

1. Lexer E. Die Verwedung der freien Knochenplastik nebst Versuchen über Gelenkversteifung und Gelenktransplanten. Langenbecks Archive für Klin. Chirung 1906;86:938 [in German].
2. Albee FH. Bone-graft surgery. Philadelphia and London: WB Saunders; 1915.
3. Adams JC. Arthrodesis of the ankle joint; experiences with the transfibular approach. J Bone Joint Surg Br 1948;30(3):506–11.
4. Leikkonen O. Astragalectomy as an ankle-stabilizing operation in infantile paralysis sequelae, with special reference to astragalectomies and total arthrodesis performed in Finland. Acta Chir Scand 1950;100(6):Suppl 152, 668–70.
5. Bingold AC. Ankle and subtalar fusion by a transarticular graft. J Bone Joint Surg Br 1956;38(4):862–70.

6. Küntscher G. Combined arthrodesis of the ankle and sub-talar joints. In: Thomas CC, editor. Practice of intramedullary nailing. Springfield (IL): Charles C Thomas; 1967. p. 207–9.
7. Stone KH, Helal B. A method of ankle stabilization. Clin Orthop Relat Res 1991;(268):102–6.
8. Dalla Paola L, Brocco E, Ceccacci T, et al. Limb salvage in Charcot foot and ankle osteomyelitis: combined use single stage/double stage of arthrodesis and external fixation. Foot Ankle Int 2009;30(11):1065–70.
9. Acosta R, Ushiba J, Cracchiolo A 3rd. The results of a primary and staged pan-talar arthrodesis and tibiotalocalcaneal arthrodesis in adult patients. Foot Ankle Int 2000;21(3):182–94.
10. Cooper PS. Complications of ankle and tibiotalocalcaneal arthrodesis. Clin Orthop Relat Res 2001;(391):33–44.
11. Hanson TW, Cracchiolo A 3rd. The use of a 95 degree blade plate and a posterior approach to achieve tibiotalocalcaneal arthrodesis. Foot Ankle Int 2002;23(8): 704–10.
12. Millett PJ, O'Malley MJ, Tolo ET, et al. Tibiotalocalcaneal fusion with a retrograde intramedullary nail: clinical and functional outcomes. Am J Orthop (Belle Mead NJ) 2002;31(9):531–6.
13. Papa J, Myerson M, Girard P. Salvage, with arthrodesis, in intractable diabetic neuropathic arthropathy of the foot and ankle. J Bone Joint Surg Am 1993; 75(7):1056–66.
14. Niinimaki TT, Klemola TM, Leppilahti JI. Tibiotalocalcaneal arthrodesis with a compressive retrograde intramedullary nail: a report of 34 consecutive patients. Foot Ankle Int 2007;28(4):431–4.
15. Wukich DK, Lowery NJ, McMillen RL, et al. Postoperative infection rates in foot and ankle surgery: a comparison of patients with and without diabetes mellitus. J Bone Joint Surg Am 2010;92(2):287–95.
16. Wukich DK, Joseph A, Ryan M, et al. Outcomes of ankle fractures in patients with uncomplicated versus complicated diabetes. Foot Ankle Int 2011;32(2):120–30.
17. Belczyk RJ, Sung W, Wukich DK. Technical tip: a simple method for proper place-ment of an intramedullary nail entry point for tibiotalocalcaneal or tibiocalcaneal Arthrodesis. Foot Ankle Online J 2008;1(9):4–11.
18. Muckley T, Ullm S, Petrovitch A, et al. Comparison of two intramedullary nails for tibiotalocalcaneal fusion: anatomic and radiographic considerations. Foot Ankle Int 2007;28(5):605–13.
19. Hammett R, Hepple S, Forster B, et al. Tibiotalocalcaneal (hindfoot) arthrodesis by retrograde intramedullary nailing using a curved locking nail. The results of 52 procedures. Foot Ankle Int 2005;26(10):810–5.
20. Quill GE. The use of second-generation intramedullary nail in the fixation of diffi-cult ankle and hindfoot arthrodeses. Am J Orthop 1999;(1-S):23–31.
21. Pochatko DJ, Smith JW, Phillips RA, et al. Anatomic structures at risk: combined subtalar and ankle arthrodesis with a retrograde intramedullary rod. Foot Ankle Int 1995;16(9):542–7.
22. McGarvey WC, Trevino SG, Baxter DE, et al. Tibiotalocalcaneal arthrodesis: anatomic and technical considerations. Foot Ankle Int 1998;19(6):363–9.
23. Budnar VM, Hepple S, Harries WG, et al. Tibiotalocalcaneal arthrodesis with a curved, interlocking, intramedullary nail. Foot Ankle Int 2010;31(12):1085–92.
24. Mann MR, Parks BG, Pak SS, et al. Tibiotalocalcaneal arthrodesis: a biomechan-ical analysis of the rotational stability of the Biomet Ankle Arthrodesis Nail. Foot Ankle Int 2001;22(9):731–3.

25. Means KR, Parks BG, Nguyen A, et al. Intramedullary nail fixation with posterior-to-anterior compared to transverse distal screw placement for tibiotalocalcaneal arthrodesis: a biomechanical investigation. Foot Ankle Int 2006;27(12):1137–42.

26. Muckley T, Hoffmeier K, Klos K, et al. Angle-stable and compressed angle-stable locking for tibiotalocalcaneal arthrodesis with retrograde intramedullary nails. Biomechanical evaluation. J Bone Joint Surg Am 2008;90(3):620–7.

27. Kaspar K, Schell H, Seebeck P, et al. Angle stable locking reduces interfragmentary movements and promotes healing after unreamed nailing. Study of a displaced osteotomy model in sheep tibiae. J Bone Joint Surg Am 2005;87(9):2028–37.

28. Klos K, Gueorguiev B, Schwieger K, et al. Comparison of calcaneal fixation of a retrograde intramedullary nail with a fixed-angle spiral blade versus a fixed-angle screw. Foot Ankle Int 2009;30(12):1212–8.

29. Berend ME, Glisson RR, Nunley JA. A biomechanical comparison of intramedullary nail and crossed lag screw fixation for tibiotalocalcaneal arthrodesis. Foot Ankle Int 1997;18(10):639–43.

30. Fleming SS, Moore TJ, Hutton WC. Biomechanical analysis of hindfoot fixation using an intramedullary rod. J South Orthop Assoc 1998;7(1):19–26.

31. Muckley T, Eichorn S, Hoffmeier K, et al. Biomechanical evaluation of primary stiffness of tibiotalocalcaneal fusion with intramedullary nails. Foot Ankle Int 2007;28(2):224–31.

32. Berson L, McGarvey WC, Clanton TO. Evaluation of compression in intramedullary hindfoot arthrodesis. Foot Ankle Int 2002;23(11):992–5.

33. Yakacki CM, Khalil HF, Dixon SA, et al. Compression forces of internal and external ankle fixation devices with simulated bone resorption. Foot Ankle Int 2010;31(1):76–85.

34. Chiodo CP, Acevedo JI, Sammarco VJ, et al. Intramedullary rod fixation compared with blade-plate-and-screw fixation for tibiotalocalcaneal arthrodesis: a biomechanical investigation. J Bone Joint Surg Am 2003;85(12):2425–8.

35. O'Neill PJ, Parks BG, Walsh R, et al. Biomechanical analysis of screw-augmented intramedullary fixation for tibiotalocalcaneal arthrodesis. Foot Ankle Int 2007;28(7):804–9.

36. O'Neill PJ, Logel KJ, Parks BG, et al. Rigidity comparison of locking plate and intramedullary fixation for tibiotalocalcaneal arthrodesis. Foot Ankle Int 2008;29(6):581–6.

37. Lee AT, Sundberg EB, Lindsey DP, et al. Biomechanical comparison of blade plate and intramedullary nail fixation for tibiocalcaneal arthrodesis. Foot Ankle Int 2010;31(2):164–71.

38. Froelich J, Idusuyi OB, Clark D, et al. Torsional stiffness of an intramedullary nail versus blade plate fixation for tibiotalocalcaneal arthrodesis: a biomechanical study. J Surg Orthop Adv 2010;19(2):109–13.

39. Alfahd U, Roth SE, Stephen D, et al. Biomechanical comparison of intramedullary nail and blade plate fixation for tibiotalocalcaneal arthrodesis. J Orthop Trauma 2005;19(10):703–8.

40. Santangelo JR, Glisson RR, Garras DN, et al. Tibiotalocalcaneal arthrodesis: a biomechanical comparison of multiplanar external fixation with intramedullary fixation. Foot Ankle Int 2008;29(9):936–41.

41. Fragomen AT, Meyers KN, Davis N, et al. A biomechanical comparison of micromotion after ankle fusion using 2 fixation techniques: intramedullary arthrodesis nail or Ilizarov external fixator. Foot Ankle Int 2008;29(3):334–41.

External Fixation Techniques for Plastic and Reconstructive Surgery of the Diabetic Foot

Ronald J. Belczyk, DPM[a],[*], Lee C. Rogers, DPM[a],
George Andros, MD[a], Dane K. Wukich, MD[b],[c],
Patrick R. Burns, DPM[a]

KEYWORDS

- Reconstructive surgery • Diabetic foot • External fixation
- Orthoplastic repair • Ilizarov circular ring fixation

Wound healing in high-risk patients with diabetes, in particular those with peripheral arterial disease and renal failure, is often lengthy due to several clinical challenges and is often fraught with complications. Clinical challenges with orthoplastic repair of the diabetic foot include simultaneous or staged management of infection, osseous deformity, early soft tissue coverage, protective off-loading, vascular issues, and medical management of diabetes and multiple comorbidities that compromise wound healing.

Techniques in plastic and reconstructive surgery of the diabetic foot continue to develop as a result of advances in external fixation. This article highlights the surgical aspect of the diabetic foot with an emphasis on the indications, advantages, technical pearls, and complications with the use of external fixation as an adjunct to plastic and reconstructive surgery of the diabetic foot.

RATIONALE FOR EXTERNAL FIXATION FOR PLASTIC AND RECONSTRUCTIVE SURGERY OF THE DIABETIC FOOT

Historically, the reconstructive ladder served as a concept of using simplest techniques and then proceeding to more complex ones. Often the simplest solution leads

[a] Amputation Prevention Center, Valley Presbyterian Hospital, 15107 Vanowen Street, Los Angeles, CA, USA
[b] Division of Foot and Ankle Surgery, Department of Orthopaedic Surgery, University of Pittsburgh School of Medicine, Pittsburgh, PA, USA
[c] Comprehensive Foot and Ankle Center, University of Pittsburgh Medical Center, Pittsburgh, PA, USA
* Corresponding author.
E-mail address: rbelczyk@hotmail.com

Clin Podiatr Med Surg 28 (2011) 649–660
doi:10.1016/j.cpm.2011.07.001
0891-8422/11/$ – see front matter © 2011 Elsevier Inc. All rights reserved.

to the safest and quickest recovery. Today, known vascularity and reliability of flaps are relied on. In many cases, however, the simplest method does not meet the requirements of a wound and the best option in some scenarios may be the more complex option. It is equally important for surgeons to be cognizant of how to protect the reconstructive efforts. Patients with diabetes have a higher risk for flap failure during the postoperative period, and the use of external fixation may increase the reliability of a complex reconstruction. Whichever soft tissue reconstructive technique is used, a protected environment is necessary to achieve primary healing. Mechanical disruption of a graft or flap during the postoperative period risks failure.

Providing an optimal environment for wound and flap healing can be challenging. Nonoperative methods for off-loading, such as frequent position changes, egg crate mattresses, Braun frames, pillows, and air or water mattresses, do not immobilize joints and are more appropriate in the prevention of wounds as opposed to surgical augmentation of the healing wound. Preconstructed devices may not be ideal in certain clinical scenarios. Although external fixation can be expensive, lengthy hospitalization and specialized beds can be cost prohibitive.[1,2] Techniques, such as total contact casting, can safely and effectively immobilize and off-load neuropathic ulcerations of the plantar forefoot and midfoot.[3] There are potential complications and limitations to consider when casting neuropathic patients. These patients often present with multiple comorbidities, such as vascular disease, edema, infection, osseous instability, and compromised soft tissue, which make casting difficult and potentially dangerous. A poorly applied cast inadequately immobilizes the extremity and potentially cause further soft tissue, skeletal, or vascular injury.[2] The presence of gross instability, polytrauma, open wounds, edema, compromised soft tissue, and/or infections may contraindicate the use of casts. For instance, some wounds secondary to diabetic Charcot neuroarthropathy potentially have gross contamination and often require simultaneous management of infection, instability, and bone loss.[2] Patients who keep the limb in a dependent position or those with cardiac or renal insufficiency experience edema, placing them at risk for complications with rigid circumferential casts. Too much or too little padding around prominences can lead to improper cast fit, resulting in cast friction–induced complications. A surgeon should provide a protective postoperative environment after a reconstructive procedure.[4] Particularly with flap surgery, plaster of Paris splints and bulky dressings hinder monitoring of flap vascularity, are uncomfortable, generally do not permit wound care, and are time consuming and painful to change.[4,5] Achieving comfort can be difficult, but patient pain should be minimal during the immediate postoperative period because inadequately managed pain can be responsible for arterial spasms.[6]

Three main advantages for the use of external fixation for plastic and reconstructive surgery of the diabetic foot include skeletal stability, soft tissue management, and assisting with wound closure techniques.

External fixation can be applied in situations when traditional methods are prohibitive or inadequate. For instance, external fixation has some advantages over circular casting in the acute setting. The benefits of external fixation include osseous stability while allowing for the damaged soft tissue to heal or demarcate, resolution of edema, and wound surveillance before definitive correction. The use of external fixation helps maintain osseous stability and limb length after acute fracture-dislocations or bone loss after staged surgical débridement of infected or avascular bone. External fixation can be used as definitive or as an adjunct to internal fixation, providing an added benefit from its load-sharing characteristics. External fixation can be used for combined osseous and soft tissue repair or it can be used independent of orthopedic injury (**Fig. 1**).

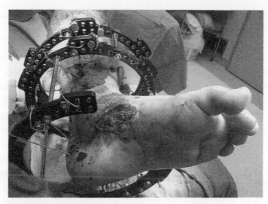

Fig. 1. This patient sustained a calcaneal fracture with an underlying compartment syndrome and underwent fasciotomy of the foot and closed reduction of the calcaneal fracture with circular ring external fixation. A split-thickness skin graft was applied to the medial compartment fasciotomy site.

When external fixation is applied solely for soft tissue protection, it is referred to as a soft tissue or an off-loading frame.[7] External fixation allows for soft tissue management in a strain-protected environment[7,8] Skin grafts applied to the foot may fail when not immobilized or off-loaded appropriately. Skin grafts are protected from weight-bearing forces if they are on the plantar aspect of foot or from range of motion from nearby joints. Local random flaps of the plantar surface may be compromised with active range of motion at the metatarsophalangeal joints or the ankle joint. Complex flaps, such as the cross-leg flaps of the lower extremity, require strict immobilization before division of the pedicle. Immobilization of the adjacent joints optimizes flap viability by minimizing intracompartment pressures in the reconstructed limb, because the position of the ankle has been shown to affect intracompartment pressures in the leg.[7,9,10] Excessive ankle dorsiflexion or plantar flexion can increase intracompartment pressures in the limb, resulting in impaired venous and arterial flow.[7] Excessive ankle motion can also cause shearing forces that may irritate the flap and vascular anastamosis.

Another advantage of the external fixator is that it permits increased surveillance of surgical incisions, open wounds, plastic reconstruction, and/or vascular repairs.[2] The ability to directly and periodically inspect the condition of the entire flap helps identify potential postoperative complications, such as infections, ischemia, venous congestion, hematoma, and trauma from inadequate immobilization or off-loading.[7] Intrinsic muscle flaps, such as the abductor digiti minimi, abductor hallucis, and flexor digitorum brevis muscle, can be used for small heel defects and the extensor digitorum brevis for the perimalleolar area. Typically, there is heavy amount of drainage postoperatively with muscle flaps, and traditional methods of cast immobilization are bulky, cumbersome, and uncomfortable during frequent dressing changes. A wound with a heavy amount of exudate presents a risk for maceration and infection if there is no access to change the dressing. Ischemia and necrosis can result from excessive tension, twisting, or kinking of a local or distant pedicle flap. The external fixator provides access and overall monitoring of the flap. Furthermore, it prevents compression of the flap.[4] A soft tissue frame has been reported to increase the flap viability rates by optimizing arteriovenous supply of to the leg and flap.[7] Immediately after a flap procedure, there may be changes in the normal vasomotor system, and the flap may be pale or slightly congested. It is possible to regulate this flow by modifying the elevation.[6] Access for repeated pulse checks after vascular repairs can help identify excessive bleeding or clotted bypass procedures.

Another advantage of the external fixator is that it reproducibly off-loads a surgeon's reconstructive efforts. It can be used to off-load definitive wound closure methods, such as skin grafting, random flaps, local or distant pedicled flaps, intrinsic muscle flaps, cross-leg flaps, or free flaps. Because the arteriovenous supply to a flap is affected by intracompartmental pressures, increased pressures by the ankle position, direct pressure on the limb, and lack of proper elevation can decrease flap inflow and promote venous congestion, thereby decreasing flap viability.[7] The soft tissue frame is an ideal limb elevator because it elevates the leg without any direct contact on the compartments of the lower extremity and also controls the position of the ankle without the use of casts, which may difficult to change in the presence of a flap.[7] The external fixator removes direct pressure from the compartments of the lower-extremity and flap and stabilizes the muscles of the leg adjacent to the flap. The reverse-flow pedicled flap should be kept slightly elevated at the level of the heart but not too high because the blood pressure decreases quickly with elevation.[6] The venous output must find its way quickly after the flap has been fixed because of true venous axis generally absent in this kind of flap. Such settlement of venous drainage needs a mechanical protection, which is provided by methods of external fixation. The use of the external fixation for 4 to 6 weeks reduces the whole region of the new vascular pattern to an acceptable strain environment.[8,11] By providing a protected environment, the healing of the flap procedure is optimized by reducing compartment pressures, off-loading the flap, and immobilizing adjacent joints.

Other considerations during the postoperative period are avoiding potential complications of strict immobilization, such as heel decubitus ulcerations and soft tissue ankle equinus contractures. The posterior heel is particularly challenging to off-load with traditional methods but the use of external fixation provides a simplistic approach to reproducibly protect this anatomic area. Temporary use of a large-frame, disposable external fixation has been safely and effectively used to prevent posterior heel soft tissue defects after polytrauma.[12] Likewise, patients with diabetes and limited mobility are at risk for developing decubitus heel ulcers. This becomes an issue after lengthy surgical times and postoperative immobilization with unprotected heels. Typical patients are those in the intensive care unit; those with polytrauma or who are sedated, geriatric, or bedridden after stroke or hip fracture repair; and those with with multiple comorbidities. Other risk factors for developing decubitus ulcerations and are commonly found in patients with diabetes include decreased sensory perception, moisture, activity, mobility, nutrition, and increased friction or shear. External fixation can help prevent heel defects in at-risk patients during this period of strict immobilization. The use of external fixation can prevent or treat acquired soft tissue contractures of the ankle. When external fixation is used after partial foot amputation procedures or free flap reconstruction of the lower extremities is performed, the foot should also be stabilized to prevent soft tissue equinus contractures of the ankle. After partial foot amputation procedures, the external fixation maintains tendon correction by limiting potential tendon retraction and contractures.[13,14]

Methods of external fixation can also assist with wound closure techniques, such as tissue expansion and closure of difficult central ray defects (described later).

PERIOPERATIVE CONSIDERATIONS

Priorities for use of external fixation in diabetic foot surgery should be complicated cases or when other simpler alternatives have failed. Patient selection is crucial to avoiding complications. Patients with psychiatric illness, gross noncompliance, or impending mortality are poor surgical candidates for external fixation. Some variables to consider include morbid obesity, lack of coordination, incapacitation of the contralateral limb, neuropathy, and spasticity, which all contribute to weight-bearing restriction and affect patient adherence to postoperative recommendations. Patients' ability to safely use assistive walking devices should be evaluated and optimized perioperatively, preferably before any elective reconstructive surgery. The first determination for limb salvage in a diabetic patient is to determine inflow. In a diabetic, selective angiography is the best method for determining inflow. If inflow is inadequate or compromised, revascularization can result in healing or promotion of wound beds suitable for simple solutions, such as skin grafts or local flaps. Multiple débridement and intravenous antibiosis may be necessary to reduce the bacterial bioburden. Once the infection has been eradicated and vascularity has been optimized, the requirements of a wound and the options for wound closure should be evaluated.

REVIEW OF FUNDAMENTAL PRINCIPLES

External fixation is an invasive surgical procedure that requires knowledge of limb anatomy for proper pin placement.[2] Surgeons should not compromise the skin or vascularity of the flap. Typical anatomic safe zones should be followed. Improper placement of half pins, transfixion pins, or fine wires may jeopardize muscles, tendons, and neurovascular structures. Other considerations that may alter the typical safe zones are patients with previous revascularization or the need to avoid placing a wire near a vascular pedicle. Typically the number of wires near the location of plastic repair should be limited and they should be placed outside the zone of plastic or vascular repair. If it is absolutely necessary to place a wire near a vessel, it is helpful to have a handheld Doppler intraoperatively to monitor for any complications of vascular impingement by external fixation pins or wire.

The authors typically limit the number of forefoot wires when possible, because this anatomic area is at increased risk for drainage and/or infection. If there is any skin tension at the pin-skin interface , this should be released intraoperatively or addressed with additional ring components or pin replacement. Compressive dressings should be used postoperatively, although this can be difficult to achieve. If forefoot plastic surgical correction is performed, it is helpful to pin the digits because movement may place additional tension along the flap. Percutaneous skeletal stabilization with Kirschner wires across the metatarsophalangeal joints or toes can be incorporated into a multiplane circular ring construct. Proper positioning of the ankle/foot in the frame is paramount, and typically the ankle is maintained at 90° to prevent equinus deformity. In select cases, slight plantar flexion of the ankle is desired to decrease skin tension of plantar rotational flap procedures. Surgeons should be knowledgeable of the principles of frame construction and specifications of multiple external fixator systems. Frames should be comfortable and allow for positioning of the lower extremity. A frame construct should accommodate a patient's individual requirements and specific plastic repair as opposed to using a one-size-fits-all frame. Considerations with maintaining patient comfort in the supine position include controlling coronal plane motion, avoiding hyperextension of the knee, avoiding any constrictive dressings, and controlling postoperative edema. Patient calf size and potential for swelling require larger constructs. Also the frame should permit visualization and access to the wound. A soft tissue offloading frame construct is generally a simpler construct, which can be constructed with the use of 2 or 3 rings and is void of dynamic components. Surgeons should understand the advantages of load-sharing fixation of both uniplanar and multiplanar frame constructs. The Ilizarov method in its traditional form and hybrid forms have greatly contributed to diabetic foot surgery with respect to Charcot foot reconstruction and off-loading of soft tissue procedures. Those patients with increased mobility requirements need increased frame stability. Some methods to increase the frame stability includes the use of olive wires, larger-diameter wires, half pins, or multiple wires; increased angulation between wires; increased ring span; and increased number of rings/hybrid components.

OFF-LOADING TECHNIQUES

An off-loading frame is typically a temporary, non–weight-bearing construct, consisting of hybrid components, including wires, pins, circular rings, and tubular bars. It combines the principles of circular ring and uniplanar frame fixation. It can be used as an adjunct to orthoplastic repair whether it is purely for soft tissue repair or supplemental to internal fixation. Iatrogenic heel ulcers result in significant additional procedures and prolonged treatment. In cases where traditional off-loading devices are difficult to apply and can interfere with proper wound care, the kickstand might provide a useful preventive solution.[1] The ideal soft tissue frame is a simple construct with minimal fixation, can be constructed according to individual patient requirements, is versatile, has one-surgeon application, is rigid, and can be modified during the postoperative period. The most common off-loading methods used by the authors includes a hybrid construct in a delta or box configuration. Another method (described later) is the use of a dummy ring for traditional Ilizarov circular ring constructs.

Hybrid Construct—Kickstand/Box Configurations

The kickstand is an extension of the hybrid construct that allows for the extremity to be off-loaded without relying on another object or without the assistance of another person. It usually consists of rods constructed in a delta configuration so that the heel is off-loaded when the patient is supine and resting the extremity over a contact surface.[1] The delta configuration means that the rods are oriented in a triangular fashion with the base oriented in a plane perpendicular to the axis of the extremity. The rods are mounted typically with pin-to-rod or rod-to-rod connecting components. The construct is designed with spacing between the flap and the device at all points to avoid direct pressure at all times.[4] The length and angle of the rods are also important considerations. Excessive pressure from contact surfaces must be avoided to prevent added morbidity from heel ulcers. The kickstand modification can be angled to prevent breakdown of the soft tissue covering involving both the posterior and plantar aspect of the heel. If the bars used are more than 15 cm, they may cause complications with hyperextension, especially when the frame does not span the knee. Relief in the popliteal area is obtained with a pillow (**Fig. 2**).[1]

The box frame is also a modification of the uniplane external fixator and can be applied relatively quickly and easily. Suspending the limb is helpful for managing a reconstructive procedure on the pressure-bearing areas, such as the posterior aspect of the ankle or leg. The frame is well tolerated by patients and permits easy wound accessibility by the nursing personnel. The authors recommend this method for only soft tissue defects that require soft tissue coverage with rotational or free tissue transfer to the posterior leg, ankle, or hindfoot.[15]

Care must be taken with the type of bed used because a kickstand could damage specialized air or water mattress (**Figs. 3–5**).[1]

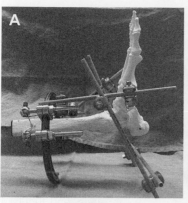
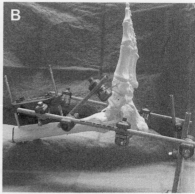

Fig. 2. Kickstand modifications on a sawbone model with varying frame configurations using (A) circular ring with fine wires and (B) half pins for supramalleolar fixation.

Circulation Ring Fixation—Dummy Ring

When a frame is used for definitive fixation, a frame construct consisting of circular rings should be considered. Circular rings permit axial micromotion, which augments fracture healing and weight bearing. It can also allow for correction of angular limb deformities with the potential for distraction and growth of new regenerate bone. When circular ring fixation is used for off-loading, the foot plate can be effective with protecting the posterior aspect of the heel. Multiple foot plates can be stacked to provide enhanced stability and increased options for pin placement, visibility and permit swelling. A simple Ilizarov frame can also be used to avoid pressure over the pedicle and the grafted donor site.[16]

A dummy ring can be a circular ring or a foot plate. It is basically an empty ring without any fixation. It is can be added to traditional Ilizarov construct to protect the plantar aspect of the foot. When used for increased frame stability, it is typically secured in the midportion of the long rods. This effectively shortens the distance between the rods. When used for off-loading purposes, this additional ring or foot plate placed inferior to the foot plate to protect the plantar aspect of the foot (Fig. 6).[17]

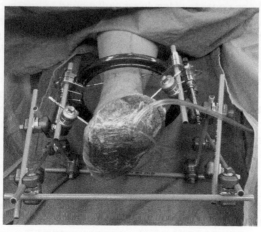

Fig. 3. A multiplanar hybrid external fixator used to off-load a skin graft on the plantar aspect of the foot.

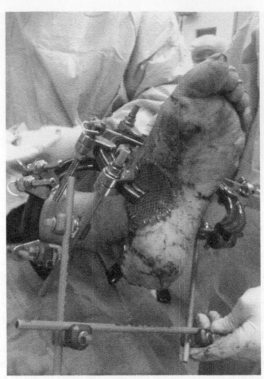

Fig. 4. Medial plantar artery island flap performed to cover a posterior heel soft tissue defect and protected with a hybrid external fixator using a kickstand modification.

TISSUE EXPANSION
Closure of Central Ray Defects

It can be difficult to manage cases when the toe and part of the metatarsal must be removed for infection or ischemia (ie, ray resection). Traditional management of central ray amputations consists of leaving a cleft wound to heal secondarily or using a split-thickness skin graft in the cleft. This results in a biomechanically unsound foot, predisposing patients to future complications. There are reports of using a cathedral-like external fixator[18,19] and a dorsal minirail fixator to close the defect and eliminate the cleft foot.[20,21] If a minirail is used, half pins are placed in the first and fifth metatarsals and the rail is attached dorsally (**Fig. 7**). The foot is manually compressed until the wound approximates. If wound approximation is not possible intraoperatively, gradual compression over 1 to 2 weeks might be necessary. Skin edges are approximated and can be sutured, including the interspace between the toes. The fixator is left in place for at least 4 weeks and the patient kept non–weight bearing or only weight bearing in a heel wedge shoe to allow the soft tissue to heal.

Skin Expansion

Forms of external fixation can also be used for skin expansion to manage large soft tissue defects. DermaClose (Wound Care Technologies, St Paul, MN, USA) uses tension line shoelaced through skin anchors implanted at the wound margins. The line is tensioned by the tension controller to 1.2 kg and locked at constant tension.

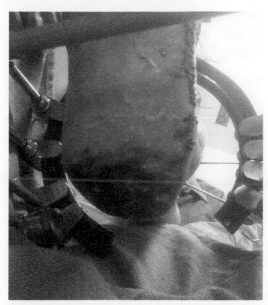

Fig. 5. Posterior heel ulceration with an abductor digiti minimi muscle flap and off-loaded with a mutliplanar external fixator.

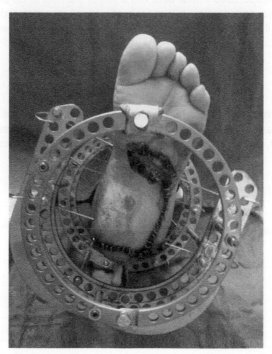

Fig. 6. A dummy ring used to off-load the plantar aspect of the foot after a rotational fasciocutaneous flap closure.

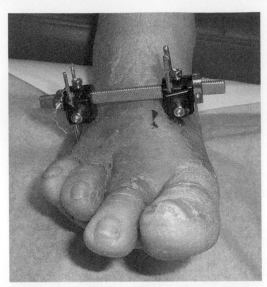

Fig. 7. A minirail external fixator (Biomet, Parsippany, NJ, USA) used to close a central ray defect after amputation.

Depending on the anatomic location, skin expands over 3 to 5 days until it is approximated (**Fig. 8**). Skin on the leg or dorsal foot expands easier and can sometimes be approximated intraoperatively. Skin near the ankle or the heel or on the medial, lateral, or plantar foot requires more time to approximate. Ideally the skin should approximate enough that it could be held with sutures under minimal tension. When approximated, the devices and anchors are removed. The margins of the wound are revised and sutures in layers.

COMPLICATIONS

Potential complications of external fixation in patients with diabetes include pin tract infection, hardware failure, iatrogenic ulcerations, scarring,[16] sepsis, fractures, muscular atrophy, and deep vein thrombosis.[7,22,23] Most of these complications are

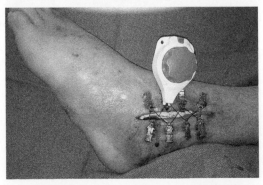

Fig. 8. A skin expansion device (DermaClose, Wound Care Technologies, St Paul, MN, USA) used to close a gaping ankle defect after incision and drainage.

minor and can be avoided with proper pin insertion, biomechanically sound constructs, decreased duration in frame, pin care, and general care of the patient (bowel, bladder, and skin care). When used for a short period of time, pin tract infections are negligible when compared with the advantages provided by external fixation.[16] Muscular atrophy during the period of immobilization is minor and is improved with physical therapy.[7] Casts are used after surgical removal of external fixation devices for period of 4 to 6 weeks to prevent fractures.

SUMMARY

The complications of diabetes are often devastating to the soft tissue and osseous structures of the foot and can require complex orthoplastic surgery. External fixation provides a protected environment by simultaneously off-loading, immobilizing joints, providing skeletal fixation, and protecting vascular repairs, permitting repeated soft tissue and vascular surveillance, wound care, and improved patient comfort, which otherwise is difficult to achieve with traditional methods. A firm grasp of fundamental principles, including proper pin placement, frame construction, and application, is of utmost importance to minimize the potential risks and complications associated with methods of external fixation in patients with diabetes.

REFERENCES

1. Castro-Aragon OE, Rapley JH, Trevino SG. The use of a kickstand modification for the prevention of heel decubitus ulcers in trauma patients with lower extremity external fixation. J Orthop Trauma 2009;23(2):145–7.
2. McHenry T, Simmons S, Alitz C, et al. Forward surgical stabilization of penetrating lower extremity fractures: circular casting versus external fixation. Mil Med 2001; 166(9):791–5.
3. Wukich DK, Motko J. Safety of total contact casting in high-risk patients with neuropathic foot ulcers. Foot Ankle Int 2004;25(8):556–60.
4. Buford GA, Trzeciak MA. A novel method for lower-extremity immobilization after free-flap reconstruction of posterior heel defects. Plast Reconstr Surg 2003; 111(2):821–4.
5. Agarwal P, Raza H. Cross-leg flap: its role in limb salvage. Indian J Orthop 2008; 42(4):439–43.
6. Masquelet A, Gilbert A. An atlas of flaps of the musculoskeletal system. United Kingdom: Informa Healthcare; 2007.
7. Sagebien CA, Rodriguez ED, Turen CH. The soft-tissue frame. Plast Reconstr Surg 2007;119(7):2137–40.
8. Klaue K. The role of external fixation in acute foot trauma. Foot Ankle Clin 2004; 9(3):583–94, x.
9. Jerosch J. Intracompartmental pressure of the anterior tibial compartment as a function of body and joint position. Biomed Tech (Berl) 1989;34(9):202–6 [in German].
10. Willy C, Gerngross H, Sterk J. Measurement of intracompartmental pressure with use of a new electronic transducer-tipped catheter system. J Bone Joint Surg Am 1999;81(2):158–68.
11. Baumeister SP, Spierer R, Erdmann D, et al. A realistic complication analysis of 70 sural artery flaps in a multimorbid patient group. Plast Reconstr Surg 2003; 112(1):129–40 [discussion: 141–22].
12. Seligson D, Douglas L. Experience with a large-frame, disposable external fixator. Orthopedics 2010;150–3.

13. Clark J, Mills JL, Armstrong DG. A method of external fixation to offload and protect the foot following reconstruction in high-risk patients: the SALSAstand. Eplasty 2009;9:e21.
14. Berkowitz MJ, Kim DH. Using an external fixation "kickstand" to prevent soft-tissue complications and facilitate wound management in traumatized extremities. Am J Orthop (Belle Mead NJ) 2008;37(3):162–4.
15. Jebson PJ, DeSilva GL, Kuzon WM Jr, et al. The box frame fixator: a technique for simultaneous fracture and free-tissue transfer management. Plast Reconstr Surg 1998;102(1):262–3.
16. Kamath JB. A simple method for pedicle protection in flap surgery for posterior heel defects. Indian J Plastic Surg 2003;36(2):104–5.
17. Nanchahal J, Pearse MF. Management of soft-tissue problems in leg trauma in conjunction with application of the Ilizarov fixator assembly. Plast Reconstr Surg 2003;111(3):1359 [author reply: 1359–60].
18. Oznur A, Tokgozoglu M. Closure of central defects of the forefoot with external fixation: a case report. J Foot Ankle Surg 2004;43(1):56–9.
19. Strauss MB, Bryant BJ, Hart JD. Forefoot narrowing with external fixation for problem cleft wounds. Foot Ankle Int 2002;23(5):433–9.
20. Bevilacqua NJ, Rogers LC, DellaCorte MP, et al. The narrowed forefoot at 1 year: an advanced approach for wound closure after central ray amputations. Clin Podiatr Med Surg 2008;25(1):127–33, viii.
21. Bernstein B, Guerin L. The use of mini external fixation in central forefoot amputations. J Foot Ankle Surg 2005;44(4):307–10.
22. Rogers LC, Bevilacqua NJ, Frykberg RG, et al. Predictors of postoperative complications of Ilizarov external ring fixators in the foot and ankle. J Foot Ankle Surg 2007;46(5):372–5.
23. Wukich DK, Belczyk RJ, Burns PR, et al. Complications encountered with circular ring fixation in persons with diabetes mellitus. Foot Ankle Int 2008;29(10):994–1000.

Advanced Foot and Ankle Fixation Techniques in Patients with Diabetes

Nicholas J. Bevilacqua, DPM[a],*, John J. Stapleton, DPM[b,c]

KEYWORDS

- Internal fixation • External fixation • Charcot foot
- Diabetic limb salvage • Foot and ankle trauma
- Revisional foot and ankle surgery • Complications

Over the past decade, there has been increasing interest in various surgical procedures and techniques for the treatment of the high-risk diabetic foot. Once considered ill advised, reconstructive foot and ankle surgery has assumed an important role in the overall management of these higher-risk patients.[1] Surgical procedures for this group have evolved from simple exostectomies to complex, corrective, reconstructive procedures. Advances in fixation techniques and technology have facilitated the evolution and complexity of procedures for diabetic foot and ankle trauma and Charcot neuroarthropathy.

The Charcot foot is a classic example of a deformity attributed to diabetes. Charcot arthropathy occurs in approximately 30% of those with peripheral neuropathy and in only 1% of the diabetic population.[2,3] Charcot arthropathy is a rapidly progressive and debilitating complication and may lead to gross deformity.[4] Early diagnosis is paramount in preventing structural collapse, and any delay in diagnosis affects outcomes. Initial management includes immobilization, offloading, and stabilization. However, in situations in which a patient presents with unstable fractures and dislocations with obvious deformity, surgical intervention may be required.

Bone mineral density is often reduced in patients with Charcot neuropathy. It is unrealistic to expect traditional internal fixation techniques alone to maintain compression across a fracture site or arthrodesis site, and fixation failure with loss of correction is common. In this situation, adjusting techniques and using supplemental fixation may enhance osseous stability. Static and dynamic external fixation constructs offer

[a] North Jersey Orthopaedic Specialists, 730 Palisade Avenue, Teaneck, NJ 07666, USA
[b] Foot and Ankle Surgery, VSAS Orthopaedics, Allentown, PA, USA
[c] Penn State College of Medicine, Hershey, PA, USA
* Corresponding author.
E-mail address: Nicholas.bevilacqua@gmail.com

Clin Podiatr Med Surg 28 (2011) 661–671
doi:10.1016/j.cpm.2011.06.007
0891-8422/11/$ – see front matter © 2011 Elsevier Inc. All rights reserved.

uniform compression and allow for placement of fine wires away from the affected bone or joint. Bridge plating with newer-generation locking plates can overcome several of the disadvantages of conventional plate fixation and provides a construct sufficiently stable to allow for osseous healing.

Recent advances in lower limb fixation methods and technologies have effectively expanded the reconstructive surgical options for the high-risk diabetic foot. Locking plate technology, external fixation, and supplemental fixation have enhanced the surgical treatment options in this high-risk population. Evolving techniques have focused on increasing the stability of fixation in poor bone quality. Sammarco[5] introduced the concept of superconstructs, in which traditional principles of fixation are abandoned to enhance stability and decrease the chance of fixation failure.

This article presents advanced techniques and current fixation constructs that are advantageous for the management of diabetic foot and ankle trauma and Charcot neuroarthropathy. Both these pathologies are often intimately related, and the fixation constructs that are needed often require sound biomechanical concepts coupled with innovative approaches to achieve bone healing and limb salvage.

BIOLOGICAL AND MECHANICAL ASPECTS OF FIXATION CHOICES

The use of internal and/or external fixation to provide osseous stability to promote bone healing among the diabetic population poses many challenges. The surgeon must understand the advantages and disadvantages of the selected fixation and recognize how the particular fixation will affect the biological cascade of events necessary for bone healing. All osteotomies, arthrodesis sites, and fractures require mechanical stability along with sufficient vascularity to create an environment that is conducive to osseous healing. In the person with diabetes and peripheral neuropathy, there is a heightened risk for fixation failure and postsurgical complications in general. There is the potential for development of Charcot neuroarthropathy and, as a result, fixation choices should be carefully considered. This patient population requires an understanding of the pathophysiology of the disease process and its inherent challenges. There is an increased need for superconstructs in this patient population, but the surgeon still has to appreciate the different effects each fixation construct has on osseous stability. Superconstructs are designed to improve stability of the fixation, and Sammarco[5] defined them as follows: (1) fusion extended beyond the zone of injury to include joints that are not affected, (2) bone resection performed to shorten the extremity to allow adequate reduction of the deformity without tension on the soft tissue envelope, (3) use of the strongest fixation device that may be tolerated by the soft tissue, and (4) fixation devices applied in a position that maximizes mechanical function. In addition, the surgeon cannot discount the importance of meticulous surgical technique and the preservation of the local vascularity to the particular bone segment.

Recent advances in techniques for the application of external fixators, particularly multiplanar, circular, and external fixators, have improved osseous stability. External fixation may maximize blood supply but may provide less osseous stability compared with internal fixation. Also, problems may arise after the external fixator is removed because continued mechanical stability is required throughout the bone healing process. Alternatively, the use of rigid compressive plates and screws provides maximum stability but may have a deleterious effect on the local blood supply and may pose a threat to the overlying soft tissues.

Locking plate technology provides a fixed-angle construct similar to an external fixator and has been called an internal-external fixator. The locking mechanism between the plate and screw head prevents toggle and back out, which may occur in osteoporotic bone. Unlike traditional plating methods, locking plates do not rely on the frictional forces between the plate and bone interface to achieve compression and stability.[6] Newer anatomically contoured locking plates allow for a limited approach or a completely percutaneous application. Locking plates have the advantage of providing improved fixation for fracture care in osteoporotic bone, and these devices provide a stable internal construct for Charcot neuroarthropathy. Current plate applications combine the benefits of compression plate fixation with the biomechanical advantages of locking plates.

Ultimately, the choice of fixation depends on many factors and should be patient specific. The surgeon should have a sound understanding of fixation principles in general, and understand the pathophysiology of the particular disease process. This is especially true when choosing the appropriate fixation construct in the person with diabetes and peripheral neuropathy. Fracture care in this high-risk population demands attention to detail. The surgeon should note the fracture pattern, consider the soft tissue envelope, and recognize the potential for the development of a Charcot neuroarthropathy. The presence of infection and/or ischemia affects fixation choice as well. In general, the choice of fixation should be determined on a case-by-case basis and certain situations may require creativity to achieve a successful outcome.

ADVANCED INTERNAL FIXATION TECHNIQUES FOR DIABETIC FOOT AND ANKLE FRACTURES

Choosing the appropriate fixation construct is critical for success in the high-risk diabetic patient. The surgeon must consider all aspects of the particular fixation construct. If using a plate, the surgeon must consider the contour and length of the plate as well as the placement, number, and type (locking vs nonlocking) of screws to be used. The physical characteristics are important to consider when choosing the appropriate internal fixation for the diabetic patient. The surgeon must be familiar with the pathology and understand which types of procedures typically require certain fixation constructs. Surgery on the diabetic foot and ankle is still evolving and an understanding of mechanically sound fixation choices for the various types of procedures performed is developing. The surgeon has to formulate an individualized treatment plan specific for each patient and tailor the fixation accordingly. For example, the surgical approach and fixation choices vary for fracture management versus arthrodesis procedures.

Although the use of locking plates is beneficial amongst this high-risk patient population, the surgeon has to appreciate the absolute stability achieved through such constructs.[7] If not properly applied, locked plates may impede bone healing.[8] This situation may occur when a fracture or arthrodesis site is stabilized with a plate and all locking screws but compression across the site is neglected. If the bone segments are slightly distracted, the absolute stability that is achieved with the locking plate may result in a nonunion. In general, locking screws should only be added after compression is obtained with nonlocking screws and should only be used when the bone is osteopenic (**Fig. 1**).

Several technical pearls have been reported for fracture care of the diabetic foot and ankle specifically regarding fixation choices. Longer plates with fewer screws can provide superior or equal strength when compared with standard compression plates using the maximum number of screws. The authors believe that the rigidity of the construct is increased with increased length of the plate (**Fig. 2**). This finding is particularly true when using medial, dorsal, and/or lateral midfoot bridge plating, often used

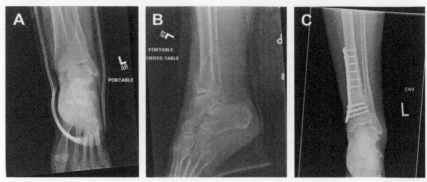

Fig. 1. Preoperative anteroposterior (*A*) and lateral (*B*) radiographs of an open distal tibia fracture. (*C*) An example of appropriate use of a locking plate for management of an open distal tibia fracture in a diabetic patient with peripheral neuropathy. Primary wound closure was performed after thorough debridement of the open fracture and lavage of the wound. Internal fixation and primary wound closure was performed because the wound was free of contamination, treated within 6 hours of the injury, and able to be closed without any tension. After the fracture was reduced, standard compression screws were used to secure the plate to the tibia both proximally and distally. Locking screws were only used for screws that did not demonstrate good cortical purchase.

for the management of isolated Lisfranc or midfoot fractures and/or dislocations. In addition, longer plates are best used for ankle and pilon fractures if the soft tissue envelope allows. When possible, the authors prefer to use a completely percutaneous plating technique for diabetic pilon fractures and, if not feasible, an attempt to extend the plate further proximally through a percutaneous approach is used to enhance stability (**Fig. 3**). A percutaneous approach combined with locking plates for the treatment of high-risk ankle and pilon fractures may decrease complications associated

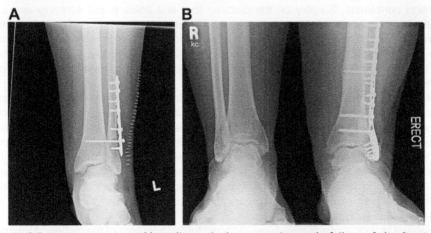

Fig. 2. (*A*) Anteroposterior ankle radiograph demonstrating early failure of the fixation. This patient had diabetes and peripheral neuropathy with loss of protective sensation and ambulated on the affected extremity, which resulted in ankle joint subluxation. (*B*) Anteroposterior view of the ankle after a revisional open reduction internal fixation was performed. The construct was further stabilized by applying a longer plate and multiple syndesmotic screws.

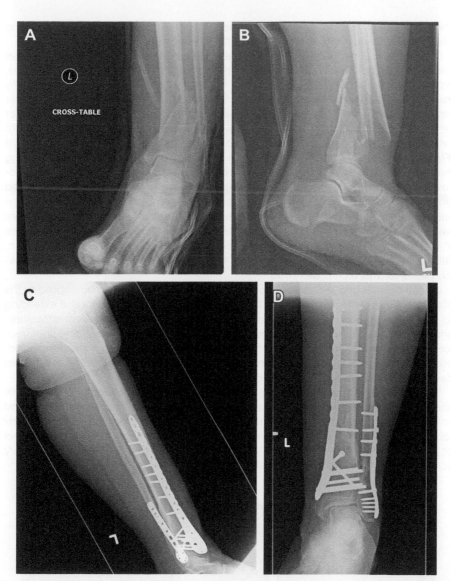

Fig. 3. (*A*) Anteroposterior and (*B*) lateral views demonstrating a severely displaced distal tibia and fibula fracture in a diabetic patient who was morbidly obese. (*C*) Anteroposterior and (*D*) lateral postoperative views demonstrating reduction of the fracture. A standard lateral approach was used in the fibula, and a percutaneous approach was used in the tibia with an extended distal tibia plate to enhance fixation and to provide absolute osseous stability.

with disruption of the soft tissue envelope.[6] However, often a completely percutaneous approach, particularly when the articular surface is severely comminuted, is not possible, and a limited open approach of the ankle joint can be performed and supplemented with longer plates extended proximally. In these cases, the appropriate contour of the plate is important to prevent wound-healing problems. The ideal plate for ankle and pilon fractures should be thin and anatomically contoured and have an appropriate bend particularly over the metaphysis of the distal tibia and the medial and lateral malleolar region to limit possible soft tissue compromise.

Bridge plating is a fixation technique that may be useful for the surgical management of diabetic midfoot fractures and/or dislocations. As with all surgical procedures, proper preoperative planning is mandatory for optimal outcome, and this is especially true when using a bridge plating technique in the midfoot. The surgeon must consider the length and arch of the column as well as the contour of the tarsal bones. For instance, when choosing a plate that spans the medial column, one must account for the anatomic contour of the arch, particularly the navicular and cuneiforms (Fig. 4). The natural arc of the cuneiforms should also be considered when placing the screws. In addition, it is important to consider the ball and socket shape of the talonavicular joint for proper screw placement. To maximize stability, plates contoured along the medial column require close attention to the precise position of the screw holes and ultimately the final screw placement. Variable angle locking plates work well for medial column bridge plating because the ideal screw placement may require 5° to 15° of angulation to appropriately accommodate the shape and arc of the arch. Otherwise, inappropriate screw placement may be seen when using fixed-angle locking plates for this technique.

Lateral column bridge plating typically requires more rotational bend applied to the plate particularly when placed along the lateral aspect of the calcaneus and extending to the fourth and fifth metatarsal bases. Despite some of the technical difficulties, bridge plating is an excellent technique for surgically managing diabetic midfoot fractures and/or dislocations. This construct can help prevent later collapse, malunion, and/or nonunion. Recently, more anatomically designed midfoot plates have been designed to account for the complex anatomy of the midfoot.

Supplemental fixation is common in the management of the neuropathic diabetic foot and ankle.[9] Supplemental fixation can be achieved in numerous ways: (1) plate and screw fixation supplemented with Kirschner wires, (2) prosyndesmotic screws with tetracortical purchase for ankle fractures,[10] (3) medial and lateral column beaming screws or Steinman pins of the midfoot,[11] (4) multiple or stacked plates, (5) intramedullary screw fixation, (6) static external fixation devices,[9,12] and (7) transarticular fixation.[13]

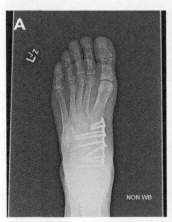
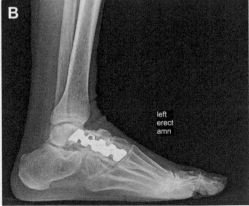

Fig. 4. (A) Anteroposterior and (B) lateral views demonstrating the of an anatomically designed midfoot plate to enhance screw purchase in the midfoot. The internal fixation in this case was used to perform a medial column fusion for a crushed midfoot in a patient with diabetes mellitus and peripheral neuropathy.

Plate and screw fixation supplemented with Kirschner wires was popularized for providing improved fixation for high-risk diabetic fibular fractures. Prosyndesmotic fixation may be used to enhance fixation among this high-risk patient population, specifically in unstable ankle fractures in patients with diabetes and neuropathy.[10,14] The use of multiple transsyndesmotic screws increases the rigidity of the entire construct. The screws are delivered through the fibular plate and are driven into the tibia purchasing all 4 cortices. The authors have expanded the role of syndesmotic screw fixation and currently recommend the use of these screws for all unstable diabetic ankle fractures, especially those with poor bone stock and/or those with comminution. The authors also use syndesmotic screw fixation for lateral malleolar fractures with an associated deltoid ligament rupture to improve stability of the ankle mortise.

Multiple or stacked plates may be used for severely comminuted distal tibia or pilon fractures (**Fig. 5**). Double plating offers increased stability and helps neutralize deforming forces that may occur over the prolonged time it takes for the osseous segments to heal. This added stability is beneficial and helps prevent loss of fracture site stability, ultimately preventing late collapse or malunion. It is important to minimize soft tissue dissection and maintain the periosteum near the fracture fragments, and only consider multiple plates if the soft tissue permits. Preserving the periosteum is paramount and the placement of the plates and screws must be meticulous. The goal is to achieve adequate fracture reduction and osseous stability while minimizing iatrogenic vascular insult to the osseous segments.

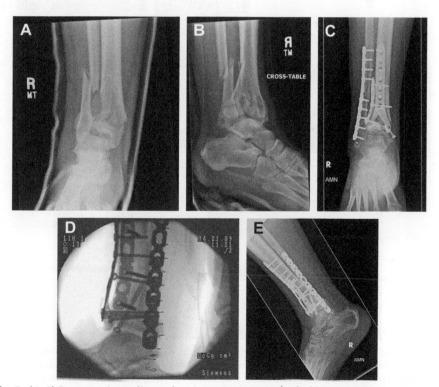

Fig. 5. (*A, B*) Preoperative radiographs of a severely comminuted tibia and fibula pilon fracture. (*C*) Anteroposterior and (*D, E*) lateral views demonstrating the use of double-plate fixation for a severely comminuted distal tibia pilon fracture.

Intramedullary nail fixation with percutaneous reduction of the fracture has the advantage of limited soft tissue disruption and preservation of the soft tissue envelope around the fracture site. This technique should be considered when managing severe diabetic distal tibia, ankle, and/or pilon fractures that are not amendable to an open procedure but require a rigid construct to maintain alignment of the foot to the leg. During the application of the intramedullary nail, the process of reaming may promote bone healing by adding autograft to the surgical site. It may also stimulate the periosteal blood supply by temporarily disturbing the endosteal blood supply. This technique may be beneficial in certain diabetic patients with coexisting peripheral neuropathy and peripheral vascular disease.

The role of external fixation is expanding, especially for the management of diabetic foot and ankle fractures.[15] The affected bone and joints may be further stabilized and better aligned, and the internal fixation construct can be supplemented with a static external fixator.[12] The authors have found the use of this technique useful for the management of fractures that are associated with severe joint dislocations (**Fig. 6**). At times, the fractures are appropriately stabilized, but alignment across the dislocated joint may not be sufficiently maintained with splinting and/or casting. This situation is typically seen with talar neck fractures (Hawkins 3 and 4), extrusions of the talus, severe open ankle dislocations, pilon fractures, and severe midfoot dislocations

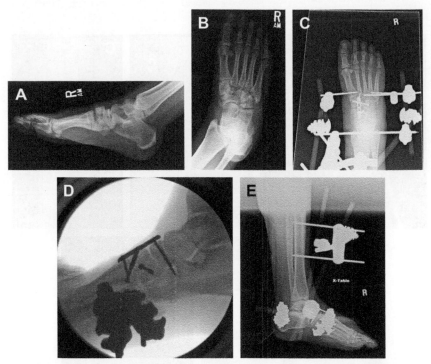

Fig. 6. (*A*) Anteroposterior and (*B*) lateral preoperative views of a severe midfoot fracture and dislocation as a result of a crush injury. The patient had a history of diabetes mellitus that was well controlled with no evidence of loss of protective sensation when examined with a 5.07 monofilament preoperatively. (*C*) Anteroposterior and lateral (*D*, *E*) radiographs demonstrate reduction by using a combination of a bridge plating technique and application of a static external fixator.

(**Fig. 7**). The supplemental use of external fixation for approximately 6 to 8 weeks often allows the necessary stabilization of the previously dislocated joints.

Transarticular fixation is an often forgotten but effective method to prevent late joint subluxation and/or to further stabilize a severe diabetic foot and ankle fracture.[13] One disadvantage of transarticular fixation is the violation and iatrogenic injury created across the articular surface. Often, this is not a major concern, particularly among individuals with diabetes and neuropathy with an insensate extremity. A second disadvantage is the fact the fixation is intra-articular. Local skin infections involving this fixation can lead to joint involvement.

ADVANCED FIXATION TECHNIQUES FOR THE CHARCOT FOOT

Charcot neuroarthropathy is perhaps the most characteristic deformity attributed to the diabetic foot, occurring in approximately 30% of individuals with peripheral neuropathy.[2] Charcot neuroarthropathy is a rapid progressive complication that often leads to gross deformity. The classic rocker-bottom deformity involving the midfoot is for many the hallmark of Charcot foot. Recognizing early bone injury is important in preserving the normal foot architecture. Early detection and treatment are associated with lower incidence of fracture and deformity and a delay in diagnosis and treatment results in progressive destruction and deformity. Initially, conservative care remains the mainstay of treatment; however, in situations in which there is significant deformity, surgical management may be required for realignment to a plantigrade extremity.

Charcot reconstruction in the setting of osteoporotic bone is frequently complicated by failure of traditional internal fixation constructs. Evolving techniques have focused

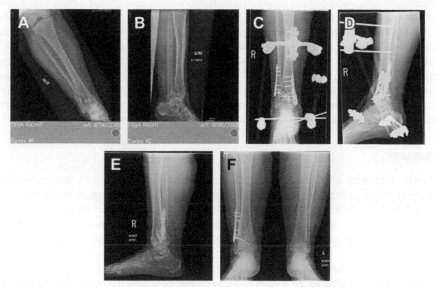

Fig. 7. (*A, B*) Preoperative radiographs showing a severely comminuted pilon fracture in a diabetic patient with peripheral neuropathy. (*C*) Anteroposterior and (*D*) lateral postoperative views demonstrating a static external fixator used to provide additional stability to a pilon fracture after an open reduction internal fixation was performed. The rationale was to prevent further lateral collapse because an extended open approach to address the lateral tibia was not performed. (*E*) Final anteroposterior and (*F*) lateral radiographs demonstrating acceptable alignment and osseous healing. The plate and screw fixation was removed 6 months postoperatively secondary to pain.

on increasing the stability of fixation by bridging the affected poor bone area and extending hardware proximally and distally.[16] This technique is often used for an extended medial column arthrodesis for Charcot midfoot deformity. After preparing the appropriate joints for fusion, a medial column plate is secured proximally to either the talus or navicular and distally to the first metatarsal. This bridging technique does not rely on fixation in the poor bone area of the midfoot. Locking plates have many desirable traits for treating Charcot neuroarthropathy; these plates have the advantage of significantly improving fixation in osteoporotic bone and are indicated in this situation.

The concept of beaming the medial and lateral columns using large-diameter screws has been described for midfoot reconstruction. These screws span the entire length of the metatarsals to the calcaneus and talus and provide compression along the columns. Advantages of this type of fixation include the limited dissection required for placement of screws, and actual placement of screws can aid in the reduction of the deformity. The screws are placed under direct visualization using fluoroscopy, and the surgeon has to account for the contour and arch of the medial and lateral columns. Screws are placed through the metatarsophalangeal joints through a plantar incision and span the entire length of the metatarsals to the calcaneus and talus. The screw heads are countersunk to the level of the distal metaphyseal-diaphyseal junction. The screws are able to resist axial loading that occurs during weight bearing. Sammarco[5] reported on a series of 22 patients who had Charcot neuroarthropathy midfoot deformity treated with a midfoot fusion using intramedullary screws for correction and fixation. All patients were considered to have successful limb salvage.

External fixation seems to be a logical choice when treating the Charcot foot and/or ankle deformity, especially in cases in which there is an associated ulceration.[17] This form of fixation, specifically multiplanar circular frames, provides uniform compression at the arthrodesis site and allows for placement of fixation away from the soft tissue defect and for continued access to the soft tissue throughout the recovery period.[18] This versatile mode of fixation may be used to provide simultaneous compression and/or distraction at different levels.[19] External fixation may also be used as supplemental fixation to internal fixation, augmenting stability.[20] Although in some ways more demanding, external fixation constructs are extremely versatile and can be tailored to each specific patient and deformity to achieve maximum stability.

SUMMARY

Diabetic foot and ankle trauma and Charcot reconstruction require a clear understanding of the pathophysiology of the disease process. The surgeon must consider patient factors, specifically peripheral neuropathy, and also factors specific to the injury or reconstruction. Appropriate preoperative planning is necessary for optimal outcome and to prevent postoperative complications. The surgeon should choose a fixation construct before embarking on a surgical procedure and understand its advantages and disadvantages for the selected procedure. The choice of fixation, whether internal, external, or a combination of the two, should be applied to provide osseous stability and account for anticipated problems commonly seen in this patient population. The surgeon should also consider the potential problems that may arise in these difficult cases.

During the last decade, advances in fixation technique and product design, especially products designed specifically for the foot and ankle, have taken place to improve the surgical outcomes in diabetic foot and ankle surgery. These advances have facilitated the evolution of treatment. The changes in technique and improvements in devices have allowed surgeons to address more complex deformities with improved outcomes. However, even with these advances, there is still a demand for further improvements as surgeons continue to manage this difficult patient population.

REFERENCES

1. Frykberg RG, Bevilacqua NJ, Habershaw G. Surgical off-loading of the diabetic foot. J Vasc Surg 2010;52:44S–58S.
2. Frykberg RG, Belczyk R. Epidemiology of the Charcot foot. Clin Podiatr Med Surg 2008;25:17–28.
3. Cofield RH, Morrison MJ, Beabout JW. Diabetic neuroarthropathy in the foot: patient characteristics and patterns of radiographic change. Foot Ankle 1983; 4:15–22.
4. Bevilacqua NJ, Bowling FL, Armstrong DG. The natural history of Charcot neuro-arthropathy. In: Frykberg R, editor. The diabetic Charcot foot: principles and management. Brooklandville (MD): Data Trace Publishing Co; 2010. p. 13.
5. Sammarco VJ. Superconstructs in the treatment of Charcot foot deformity: plantar plating, locked plating, and axial screw fixation. Foot Ankle Clin 2009;14:393–407.
6. Lee T, Blitz NM, Rush SM. Percutaneous contoured locking plate fixation of the pilon fracture: surgical technique. J Foot Ankle Surg 2008;47:598–602.
7. O'Neill PJ, Logel KJ, Parks BG, et al. Rigidity comparison of locking plate and intra-medullary fixation for tibiotalocalcaneal arthrodesis. Foot Ankle Int 2008;29:581–6.
8. Bottlang M, Lesser M, Koerber J, et al. Far cortical locking can improve healing of fractures stabilized with locking plates. J Bone Joint Surg Am 2010;92:1652–60.
9. Wukich DK, Kline AJ. The management of ankle fractures in patients with diabetes. J Bone Joint Surg Am 2008;90:1570–8.
10. Perry MD, Taranow WS, Manoli A 2nd, et al. Salvage of failed neuropathic ankle fractures: use of large-fragment fibular plating and multiple syndesmotic screws. J Surg Orthop Adv 2005;14:85–91.
11. Sammarco VJ, Sammarco GJ, Walker EW Jr, et al. Midtarsal arthrodesis in the treatment of Charcot midfoot arthropathy. J Bone Joint Surg Am 2009;91:80–91.
12. Marin LE, Wukich DK, Zgonis T. The surgical management of high- and low-energy tibial plafond fractures: a combination of internal and external fixation devices. Clin Podiatr Med Surg 2006;23:423–44, vii.
13. Jani MM, Ricci WM, Borrelli J Jr, et al. A protocol for treatment of unstable ankle fractures using transarticular fixation in patients with diabetes mellitus and loss of protective sensibility. Foot Ankle Int 2003;24:838–44.
14. Schon LC, Marks RM. The management of neuroarthropathic fracture-dislocations in the diabetic patient. Orthop Clin North Am 1995;26:375–92.
15. Prisk VR, Wukich DK. Ankle fractures in diabetics. Foot Ankle Clin 2006;11:849–63.
16. Zgonis T, Roukis TS, Lamm BM. Charcot foot and ankle reconstruction: current thinking and surgical approaches. Clin Podiatr Med Surg 2007;24:505–17, ix.
17. Bevilacqua NJ, Rogers LC. Surgical management of Charcot midfoot deformities. Clin Podiatr Med Surg 2008;25:81–94.
18. Zgonis T, Stapleton JJ, Jeffries LC, et al. Surgical treatment of Charcot neuropathy. AORN J 2008;87:971–86 [quiz: 987–90].
19. Zgonis T, Stapleton JJ, Roukis TS. Use of circular external fixation for combined subtalar joint fusion and ankle distraction. Clin Podiatr Med Surg 2008;25:745–53, xi.
20. Stapleton JJ, Belczyk R, Zgonis T. Revisional Charcot foot and ankle surgery. Clin Podiatr Med Surg 2009;26:127–39.

Internal Fixation Techniques for Midfoot Charcot Neuroarthropathy in Patients with Diabetes

Brandon E. Crim, DPM[a], Nicholas J. Lowery, DPM[b],*,
Dane K. Wukich, MD[c]

KEYWORDS

• Charcot neuropathic osteoarthropathy
• Internal fixation techniques • Diabetes • Treatment

Charcot neuropathic osteoarthropathy (CN) of the foot and ankle is a poorly understood destructive process that poses a great clinical challenge to foot and ankle specialists. Neuropathic fractures or dislocations in the foot and ankle predispose patients to increased morbidity, premature mortality, and can greatly decrease quality of life.[1] Early recognition and treatment of CN is imperative to prevent the development of permanent deformities.[2]

Primary treatment of acute CN is largely nonoperative using off-loading techniques, such as total contact casting, bracing, and Charcot restraint orthotic walker devices. When nonoperative measures fail to control deformity and prevent ulceration, surgical management may be warranted. The purpose of this article is to review the history, cause, and classification of CN and to discuss commonly used internal fixation techniques and their indications.

HISTORY OF CHARCOT NEUROPATHIC OSTEOARTHROPATHY

CN of the foot and ankle is a disease process that, even after 300 years, remains enigmatic. Charcot disease has been associated with leprosy, toxic exposure, syringomyelia, poliomyelitis, rheumatoid arthritis, multiple sclerosis, congenital neuropathy,

[a] University of Pittsburgh Medical Center, Pittsburgh, PA, USA
[b] The Wound and Skin Healing Center at Washington Hospital, Washington, PA, USA
[c] Department of Orthopaedic Surgery, University of Pittsburgh Medical Center, Pittsburgh, PA, USA
* Corresponding author.
E-mail address: lowerynj@upmc.edu

Clin Podiatr Med Surg 28 (2011) 673–685
doi:10.1016/j.cpm.2011.08.003   podiatric.theclinics.com
0891-8422/11/$ – see front matter © 2011 Elsevier Inc. All rights reserved.

traumatic injury, and diabetes.[3–5] Sir William Musgrave was the first to report on neuropathic arthritis in 1703 in patients with venereal disease.[3,6] In 1831, Mitchell described a relationship between caries (tuberculosis) of the spinal cord and hot, swollen, asymmetrical joints, which he labeled "rheumatism of the lower extremities."[7] In 1868, Jean Martin Charcot described the neuropathic component of the disease process in patients with tertiary syphilis.[8] He recognized the importance of the discoveries of previous investigators and described a hypertrophic process of destructive arthritis. Fifteen years later, Charcot and Fere published their observations in *The Short Bones and Small Joints of the Foot*.[9] Theses findings gained international fame at the Seventh International Medical Congress in London where Sir James Paget coined the term "Charcot's disease." In 1936, Jordan provided a link between neuropathic osteoarthropathy and diabetes mellitus.[10] Currently, diabetes mellitus is the leading cause of CN, with a prevalence ranging from 0.08% to 7.5% of patients with diabetese.[5] The true prevalence of CN is unknown because many patients remain undiagnosed.

CLASSIFICATION OF CHARCOT

Eichenholtz's landmark monograph, published in 1966, classified Charcot arthropathy based on radiographic appearance and physiologic course.[11] The disease process was classified into 3 separate but linear stages: development, coalescence, and reconstructive stages. Shibata and colleagues[12] later modified this classification to include a precursor to stage 1. This stage has been labeled Charcot in situ, prestage 1, or most commonly stage 0 Charcot.[13–15] Frequently misdiagnosed as gout, cellulitis, or deep vein thrombosis, stage 0 CN begins with an initial insult to the neuropathic foot and ankle resulting in erythema, edema, warmth, and often pain.[12,16] This presentation is most commonly unilateral, although bilateral cases have been reported in approximately 10% of patients.[17] Identification and intervention during this early, prodromal stage may prevent the progression and complications associated with Charcot.[2] Stage 1 (development) continues with redness, swelling, warmth, and has the radiographic appearance of bony debris, fragmentation, subluxations, dislocations, and periarticular fragmentation.[11] Stage 2 (coalescence) demonstrates decreased erythema, edema, and warmth, with radiographic signs of healing fracture fragments and the appearance of bony sclerosis. Stage 3 (remodeling) demonstrates final consolidation of fracture fragments with the absence of the clinical signs present in stage 0 and 1.

Several investigators have described the anatomic patterns of involvement in CN based on location. Sanders and Frykberg classified 5 anatomic patterns (**Table 1**): pattern 1 forefoot (15%), pattern 2 tarsometatarsal joints (40%), pattern 3 midtarsal

Table 1		
Anatomic classification system for Charcot neuroarthropathy according to Sanders and Frykberg		
Pattern	**Location**	**Percentage of Cases**
Pattern I	Forefoot (Metatarsophalangeal joint/Interphalangeal joint)	15
Pattern II	Tarsometatarsal joints	40
Pattern III	Naviculocuneiform, talonavicular, calcaneocuboid joints	30
Pattern IV	Talocrural, subtalar joints	10
Pattern V	Calcaneus	5

Data from Sanders L, Frykberg RG. Diabetic neuropathic osteoarthropathy: the Charcot foot. In: Frykberg RG, editor. The high risk foot in diabetes mellitus. New York: Churchill Livingstone; 1991. p. 297–338.

joints (30%), pattern 4 ankle and subtalar joints (10%), pattern 5 calcaneus (5%).[18] More than one pattern of destruction can coexist. For example, it is common to observe tarsometatarsal involvement with subsequent navicular destruction.

In 1993, Brodsky described 4 areas of destruction in Charcot neuroarthropathy (Table 2).[19] Type 1 includes the midfoot and is the most common location, affecting approximately 60% of patients with CN. Type 2 involves the rear foot triple joint complex, including the subtalar, talonavicular, and calcaneocuboid joints, affecting 20% to 25% of patients. Type 3 is divided into 2 subtypes: subtype A affects the tibiotalar joint and subtype B affects the posterior calcaneus. The incidence of these subtypes is 9% and 2%, respectively. Brodsky did not include the forefoot in his classification system, an anatomic region that accounts for approximately 15% of cases according to Sanders and Frykberg.[18]

Because of the increased incidence of midfoot and medial column involvement, Schon and colleagues[20] further classified these anatomic areas. Based on the examination of 3 standard radiographic views of 131 feet in 109 patients, 4 patterns were devised for midfoot and medial column involvement. The Lisfranc pattern includes the breakdown of the first 3 tarsometatarsal joints, with progression to the fourth and fifth tarsometatarsal joints in more severe cases. The naviculocuneiform pattern describes involvement of the more proximal and medial naviculocuneiform joint. The perinavicular pattern and transverse tarsal pattern describe involvement of their respective joints.

The focus of this article is on those with midfoot CN. These patients frequently present with plantar ulceration at the apex of their deformity, often with a rocker-bottom–type appearance. Although there are typically multiple areas of deformity, including equinus, the treatment of midfoot dislocation and subluxation are discussed here (Fig. 1).

Certain proinflammatory cytokines have been linked to mediators of bone resorption. In a study of CN reactive bone, Baumhauer and colleagues[21] demonstrated an increase in osteoclasts when compared with osteoblast. This disproportionate increase in osteoclasts results in localized decreased bone mineral density (BMD) a factor that may play an important role in the pathogenesis of CN. In 2004, Herbst and colleagues[22] separated the pattern of Charcot in the foot and ankle into 3 distinctive groups: fracture, dislocation, and combined fracture dislocation. They concluded that the pattern of Charcot may be based on BMD. Although the BMD of all patients with Charcot may not be pathologic, those with the fracture pattern had a significantly lower BMD. They concluded that the fracture pattern may be based on a decreased BMD, whereas the dislocation and combined pattern will be present in patients with a more normalized BMD. The quality of bone is an important factor when deciding

Table 2		
Anatomic classification system for Charcot neuroarthropathy according to Brodsky		
Type	Location	Percentage of Cases
Type 1	Midfoot (tarsometatarsal, naviculocuneiform joints)	60
Type 2	Hindfoot (subtalar, calcaneocuboid, talonavicular joints)	25
Type 3A	Ankle joint	10
Type 3B	Posterlor calcaneus	5

Data from Brodsky JW, Rouse AM. Exostectomy for symptomatic bony prominences in diabetic Charcot feet. Clin Orthop Relat Res 1993;(296):21–6.

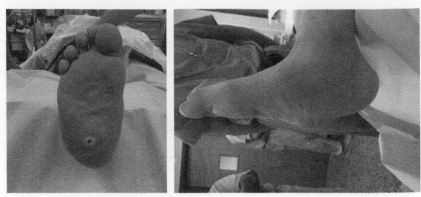

Fig. 1. Clinical examples of midfoot Charcot rocker-bottom foot with ulceration.

what type of fixation construct will be used, and the presentation of the deformity may give a clinical clue as to the bone quality. Vitamin D and renal disease most likely play a role as well, although it is not fully understood.

INDICATIONS FOR SURGERY

High-level evidence supporting the basis of surgical therapies in the treatment of patients with Charcot arthropathy is lacking.[23] The difficulty of structuring a blinded, prospective, randomized study in a surgical specialty limits the availability of high-level evidence, and the relatively low prevalence of Charcot arthropathy restricts the number of patients per study. Wukich and colleagues[23,24] performed a MEDLINE search and identified 499 articles on the subject of the surgical management of patients with diabetes and CN.

The current knowledge base for operative management of CN is based on approximately 1100 patients who have been reported in the literature between 1960 and 2009. This number may be overestimated because some investigators may have reported data on the same patients in separate articles. As hypothesized, the surgical management of Charcot neuroarthropathy is based on retrospective case series, and no prospective, randomized studies have been performed to date.

Patients with CN may present for treatment at any stage of the disease, but the common reasons for seeking medical consultation include mild to moderate pain, severe edema of the foot or ankle, and an inability to put on shoes.[25] Pain, in a patient with an insensate foot, should be an indicator of a much larger problem, such as deep infection. It is imperative to investigate for any previous history of infections or ulcerations to rule out a recurring acute or chronic infection. Systemic signs of infection include leukocytosis, elevated C-reactive protein and erythrocyte sedimentation rate levels, and recent unexplained hyperglycemia, although patients with diabetes may have immunopathy and not mount a normal inflammatory response.[23,26,27] Osteomyelitis should be considered in patients with a history of ulceration, specifically when an ulcer probes to the bone. The diagnosis of osteomyelitis in patients with diabetic CN can be difficult because of unreliable clinical signs and laboratory values and similar radiographic changes.[28] Signs of inflammation may be absent in up to two-thirds of ulcers with histopathologic evidence of osteomyelitis.[29] It is important to correlate clinical findings, laboratory values, and advanced imaging studies to rule out infection (**Fig. 2**).

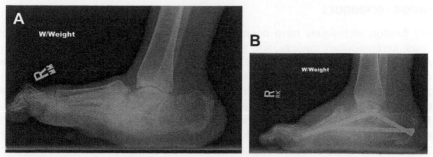

Fig. 2. Preoperative (*A*) and postoperative (*B*) lateral radiographs of midfoot Charcot neuro-arthropathy. Preoperative radiograph demonstrates a negative Meary angle, which is a risk factor for ulceration. Postoperative radiograph demonstrates a reconstructed Meary angle with the use of an intramedullary bolt. Note the equinus deformity in the preoperative radiograph evident by the decreased calcaneal inclination angle.

The indications for surgical reconstruction of the midfoot in CN includes recurring ulceration, joint instability, pain associated with malalignment, offending exostoses, and potential skin complications from the inability to brace or from a nonplantigrade foot.[30] The long-term goals for operative and nonoperative treatment are to achieve a stable, plantigrade functional foot that is resistant to ulceration; prevent amputation; and improve performance in activities of daily living.[31] Surgical reconstruction for the deformed foot and ankle has historically been recommended after all nonoperative measures to prevent further breakdown have been exhausted.[32]

Bevan and Tomlinson[33] studied 24 feet in 19 patients to identify a radiographic predictor for ulceration in a group of patients with CN. The results of the study showed that the lateral talar-first metatarsal angle (Meary angle) showed a statistically significant association with a pathologic skin condition. Patients with a lateral talar-first metatarsal angle of greater than negative 27 degrees correlated with current or impending ulceration, This finding may be an indication for surgical intervention (**Fig. 3**).

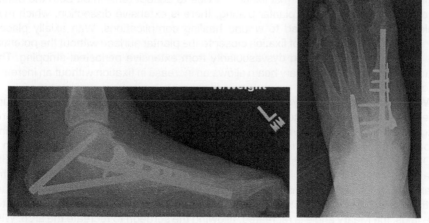

Fig. 3. Correction of midfoot Charcot deformity with the use of intramedullary bolt fixation. Note the adjunctive use of a medially placed locking plate to aide in frontal plane stability.

FIXATION TECHNIQUES

Many fixation techniques have been described in the literature, including plates, screws, intramedullary devices, and external fixation. No consensus in the literature has been reached regarding optimal fixation techniques because none have been proven to be superior. Recent advances in internal fixation techniques, such as locking plate technology, solid fixation bolts, and intramedullary superconstructs, have provided encouraging options in patients undergoing surgical management.

Because of the inherent nature of bony destruction and disorganization of CN, the surgical reconstruction of midfoot deformities is complicated. Standard fixation techniques using obliquely oriented lag screws are often inadequate because of the bony changes that accompany the Charcot process.[31] Poor bone quality and vascularity, neuropathy, and impaired nutrition are intrinsic variables that may be associated with delayed osseous healing. The need for long periods of strict non–weight bearing during the postoperative period is often challenging in this patient population. Patients with diabetes often have a difficult time with non–weight bearing secondary to neuropathy, obesity, and poor flexibility.

The need for more advantageous fixation has led to the term "superconstructs" when dealing with midfoot Charcot.[31] A superconstruct is defined by 4 factors: (1) fusion is extended beyond the zone of injury to include joints that are not affected to improve fixation, (2) bone resection is performed to shorten the extremity to allow for adequate reduction of deformity without undue tension on the soft tissue envelope, (3) the strongest device is used that can be tolerated by the soft tissue envelope, and (4) the devices are applied in a position that maximizes mechanical function. Superconstructs are warranted in cases that have a high likelihood for failure and are appropriate in the setting of dysvascular bone, bone loss, deformity correction, severe osteoporosis, and in patients with multiple medical comorbidities that can lead to delayed healing.[31] With the use of these techniques, multiple joints are fused to correct the deformity, with large spanning fixation. Sammarco[31] identified 3 superconstructs in the reconstruction of midfoot Charcot deformity: plantar plating, locking plate technology, and axial screw fixation.[31,34]

Axial screw placement, or intramedullary beaming, is the placement of a solid or cannulated screw within the medullary cavity of multiple bones to fixate the deformity. There are multiple benefits to intramedullary beaming. The placement of an intramedullary screw allows the internal fixation device to accept tension on both the dorsal and plantar surfaces. With plantar plating, there is extensive dissection, which may delay bone healing and lead to wound healing complications. With axially placed screws, there is the benefit of fixation closer to the plantar surface without the potential for wound complication and dysvascularity from extensive periosteal stripping. The placement of an intramedullary beam allows an increase in fixation without an increase in dissection.

With any type of deformity correction, it is important to have a systematic, reproducible way of reducing the abnormal extremity. The concept of the center of rotation and angulation (CORA) has provided guidelines and assists in making deformity planning more reproducible.[35] With midfoot Charcot deformity, there is usually more than 1 CORA. The most obvious is the CORA formed by the plantarflexed talus along with the midfoot sag within the sagittal plane. It is important to remember that these are triplanar deformities, with transverse and frontal plane involvement. By placing a beam within the first metatarsal across the medial column and inserting it proximally to enter the talus, the Meary angle is recreated, allowing the surgeon to recreate the arch. With this technique, an intramedullary screw can be placed along the medial column following joint preparation to perform an arthrodesis procedure. Early attempts at placement of intramedullary screw fixation failed because of the lack of joint preparation for arthrodesis of midfoot joints. If there is lateral column involvement, axially placed screws can be placed within the medial and lateral columns. With the additional subtalar joint fusion, both columns of the foot are no longer independent and work together in a tripod alignment to share the load. The midfoot beam will resist forces within the sagittal and transverse planes because of the placement within the intramedullary cavity of the bone. Depending on the fixation device, the threads of the screw may only engage the proximal bones, most commonly the talus. This placement means the distal bones only have contact with the shank of the screw, and this can lead to frontal plane rotation. The addition of a locking plate will resist frontal plane rotation and mimics a static screw in an intramedullary rod (**Fig. 4**).[36]

There are many complications with any arthrodesis procedure. Within the Charcot literature, nonunion and wound healing problems are complications that are often

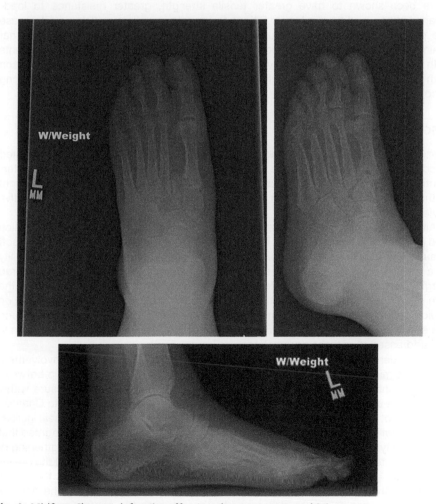

Fig. 4. Midfoot Charcot deformity affecting the tarsometatarsal joint.

addressed. The placement of a solid midfoot bolt has the benefit of increased strength as compared with cannulated screws, although it is technically more difficult to perform. The solid bolt can be inserted following the removal of a guidewire, which is used to verify proper placement and for drilling. With the placement of midfoot bolts, the construct may be strong enough to withstand the force imparted on it even in the face of nonunion. Intramedullary placement of axial screws has an advantage in the face of wound dehiscence. Because of the placement of the beam within the medullary cavity of the bone, the surrounding soft tissue and bone act as a biologic barrier protecting the hardware from the outside environment.

Comparisons between stainless steel and titanium screws can be found within the literature. Titanium implants are excellent for permanent fixation because of their corrosion resistance, adherence to bone and soft tissue, absence of allergic response, and overall good biocompatibility. The major limitation of titanium screws in a Charcot foot reconstruction is its long-term durability with a reduced tensile strength when compared with stainless steel.[37,38] Stainless steel fixation devices have been shown to have greater tensile strength, greater resistance to load-bearing stress, and have a longer fatigue failure rate over time, which may decrease the potential for implant failure or broken hardware.[39] It is for these reasons that stainless steel fixation screws should be used in midfoot reconstruction in patients with CN.[38] Solid fixation bolts have the added advantage of strength in comparison with cannulated screws, although they may be more challenging to place during reconstruction.

DISCUSSION

Pinzur and colleagues[40,41] reported that 60% of patients with midfoot CN were treated successfully without surgery. The remaining 40% of patients required surgical intervention, most commonly a triple arthrodesis to create a more plantigrade foot. Eight of the 147 (5.4%) patients went on to amputation within the 1 year of this retrospective review.

Although the aforementioned classification systems are based on anatomic location and bony pathologic conditions, it is important to recognize the involvement of the soft tissues. Brink and colleagues[42] discussed ligamentous laxity and soft tissue instability in a case of talar dislocation in a patient with Charcot foot. The patient required surgical correction, which included a triple arthrodesis. This article highlights the role of soft tissue failure. Although fractures and dislocations can be clearly seen on radiographs, it is important to remember that there is failure on multiple levels, and the soft tissues must be addressed when correcting this deformity.[42] Arthrodesis in CN addresses all of these parameters.

The influence of the Achilles tendon is a clear example of soft tissue involvement within the midfoot collapse. There is controversy on the causal relationship between equinus contracture and Charcot collapse.[30] Equinus increases the pressure within the midfoot and forefoot; however, not all patients with equinus progress to Charcot. With midfoot collapse and subsequent rocker-bottom deformity, the calcaneal inclination angle will decrease and often become a negative value. In general, it is agreed that equinus plays some role in the deformity, and reconstruction includes lengthening of the Achilles tendon or gastrocnemius aponeurosis. In theory, lengthening of the posterior muscle group increases the calcaneal inclination angle and relieves the stress placed on the midfoot joints.[30] It has been shown that lengthening of the Achilles tendon decreases its power, decreases the pressure on the midfoot and forefoot, and increases the available dorsiflexion at the ankle joint.

CASE PRESENTATION

A 67-year-old woman presented to the authors' institution with erythema and edema to her left foot. She was previously seen by her primary care physician approximately 1 month before her visit. She was being treated for cellulitis and was placed on 3 different courses of antibiotics without resolution of her symptoms. She complained of an insidious onset of redness, swelling, and pain in her left midfoot, although she did not recall any traumatic injury or inciting incident. She had a history Type 2 diabetes mellitus for 2 years and associated peripheral neuropathy. Before this visit she was never offloaded. Although she is neuropathic, she did complain of pain and she noticed that her left foot now looks different. She denies any constitutional symptoms, such as nausea, vomiting, fevers, or increases in her blood sugar. She presented to the foot and ankle clinic for a second opinion for her left foot.

On physical examination, her pedal pulses were palpable. Her neurologic examination was grossly abnormal, including absent sensation with the Semmes Weinstein monofilament, absent vibratory sensation with the 128 Hz tuning fork, and absent deep tendon reflexes at the level of the ankle. Digital contractures were also present bilaterally, consistent with intrinsic muscle atrophy secondary to neuropathy. Her left foot seemed mildly edematous with some local erythema around the first and second tarsometatarsal joints. The midfoot seemed abducted in the transverse plane. She had tenderness on palpation of the first and second tarsometatarsal joints of the left foot, and there was also crepitus and instability noted. Her skin was intact with no sign of ulceration or preulcerative lesions. She also had a large dorsal prominence at the first tarsometatarsal joint. During her clinic evaluation, her left foot was elevated and the erythema improved significantly, suggesting against the diagnosis of cellulitis. She also demonstrated a gastrocnemius-soleus equinus contracture of her left lower extremity.

Radiographs of her left foot demonstrated subluxation of the first and second tarsometatarsal joints, with changes suggestive of CN. The first metatarsal had subluxation medially and dorsally, and the second metatarsal had subluxation laterally and dorsally from the intermediate cuneiform. Swelling of the soft tissues was also noted. Magnetic resonance imaging demonstrated increased signal intensity on T2-weighted images throughout the midfoot, with confirmation of first and second tarsometatarsal joint subluxation (**Fig. 5**).

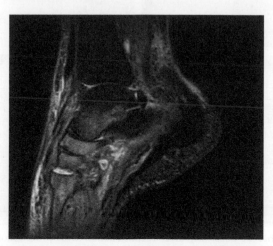

Fig. 5. Increased signal intensity in the midfoot consistent with Charcot neuroarthropathy.

Laboratory studies were also ordered to assist in the differentiation between infection and Charcot. Her C-reactive protein was 0.8, and her sedimentation rate was 15. Her white blood cell count was 7200 (**Fig. 6**).

Initially, the patient was treated with total contact cast after the diagnosis of Eichenholtz stage 1 CN was made. After resolution of the erythema and edema, she continued to complain of pain associated with her midfoot deformity. She could not ambulate despite being treated with orthotics and extra depth shoes. Her American Orthopaedic Foot and Ankle score at this point was 13, demonstrating severe functional impairment. At this point the decision was made to proceed with reconstruction of her CN deformity. The surgical plan included open reduction and primary fusion of her first and second tarsometatarsal joints using intramedullary fixation for the medial

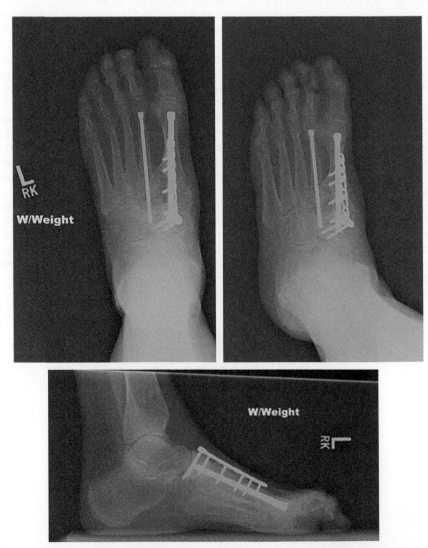

Fig. 6. Midfoot Charcot deformity after reconstruction with intramedullary fixation and locking plate.

column and the second ray and supplemental fixation consisting of a dorsal locking plate. An incision was made over the first and second tarsometatarsal joint, and her dislocation was immediately evident. The joints were reduced and the articular cartilage was denuded. Autogenous bone graft was harvested from the distal tibia and placed into the fusion sites. A 6.5-mm headless screw was then placed in retrograde fashion across the first tarsometatarsal joint and a 4.5-mm headless screw was placed in retrograde fashion across the second tarsometatarsal joint. A supplemental locking plate was then placed dorsally to achieve additional stability. Closure was performed in typical layers and the patient was placed into a Jones compression splint with plaster.

Her postoperative course included 8 weeks in a short-leg non–weight bearing cast followed by 8 weeks of protected weight bearing. Postoperative radiographs demonstrate progressive fusion across the first and second tarsometatarsal joints with all hardware intact. Her talar-first metatarsal angle is within normal limits and her foot is plantigrade. Her pain has decreased and she has been able to transition into regular shoes.

REFERENCES

1. Dhawan V, Spratt KF, Pinzur MS, et al. Reliability of AOFAS diabetic foot questionnaire in Charcot arthropathy: stability, internal consistency, and measurable difference. Foot Ankle Int 2005;26(9):717–31.
2. Wukich DK, Sung W, Wipf SA, et al. The consequences of complacency: managing the effects of unrecognized Charcot feet. Diabet Med 2010;28(2): 195–8.
3. Gupta R. A short history of neuropathic arthropathy. Clin Orthop Relat Res 1993; 296:43–9.
4. Johnson JT. Neuropathic fractures and joint injuries. Pathogenesis and rationale of prevention and treatment. J Bone Joint Surg Am 1967;49(1):1–30.
5. Sanders L, Frykberg RG. The Charcot foot (Pied de Charcot). In: Bowker JH, Pfeifer MA, editors. Levin and O'Neal's The diabetic foot. Philidelphia: Mosby Elsevier; 2007. p. 257–83.
6. Armstrong DG, Peters EJ. Charcot's arthropathy of the foot. J Am Podiatr Med Assoc 2002;92(7):390–4.
7. Mitchell JK. On a new practice in acute and chronic rheumatism. Am J Med Sci 1831;8:55–64.
8. Charcot JM. Sur quelques arthropathies qui paraissent dependre d'une lesion du cerveau ou de la moelle epinere. Archive de Physiologie Normale Pathologique 1868;1:161–78 [in French].
9. Charcot JM, Fere C. Affections Osseuses et articulares du pied chez les tabiteques. Archives de neurologie 1883;6:305–19 [in French].
10. Jordan W. Neuritic manifestations in diabetes mellitus. Arch Intern Med 1936;57: 307–66.
11. Eichenholtz S. Charcot joints. Charles C. Thomas; 1966. p. 3–8.
12. Shibata T, Tada K, Hashizume C. The results of arthrodesis of the ankle for leprotic neuroarthropathy. J Bone Joint Surg Am 1990;72(5):749–56.
13. Schon LC, Marks RM. The management of neuroarthropathic fracture-dislocations in the diabetic patient. Orthop Clin North Am 1995;26(2):375–92.
14. Sella EJ, Barrette C. Staging of Charcot neuroarthropathy along the medial column of the foot in the diabetic patient. J Foot Ankle Surg 1999;38(1):34–40.

15. Yu GV, Hudson JR. Evaluation and treatment of stage 0 Charcot's neuroarthrop-
    athy of the foot and ankle. J Am Podiatr Med Assoc 2002;92(4):210–20.
16. Chantelau E. The perils of procrastination: effects of early vs. delayed detec-
    tion and treatment of incipient Charcot fracture. Diabet Med 2005;22(12):
    1707–12.
17. Saltzman CL, Hagy ML, Zimmerman B, et al. How effective is intensive nonoper-
    ative initial treatment of patients with diabetes and Charcot arthropathy of the
    feet? Clin Orthop Relat Res 2005;435:185–90.
18. Sanders L, Frykberg RG. Diabetic neuropathic osteoarthropathy: the Charcot
    foot. In: Frykberg RG, editor. The high risk foot in diabetes mellitus. New York:
    Churchill Livingstone; 1991. p. 297–338.
19. Brodsky JW, Rouse AM. Exostectomy for symptomatic bony prominences in dia-
    betic Charcot feet. Clin Orthop Relat Res 1993;296:21–6.
20. Schon LC, Easley ME, Weinfeld SB. Charcot neuroarthropathy of the foot and
    ankle. Clin Orthop Relat Res 1998;349:116–31.
21. Baumhauer JF, O'Keefe RJ, Schon LC, et al. Cytokine-induced osteoclastic bone
    resorption in Charcot arthropathy: an immunohistochemical study. Foot Ankle Int
    2006;27(10):797–800.
22. Herbst SA, Jones KB, Saltzman CL. Pattern of diabetic neuropathic arthropathy
    associated with the peripheral bone mineral density. J Bone Joint Surg Br
    2004;86(3):378–83.
23. Wukich DK, Sung W. Charcot arthropathy of the foot and ankle: modern concepts
    and management review. J Diabetes Complications 2009;23(6):409–26.
24. Wukich DK, Lowery NJ, Woods J, et al. Surgical management of diabetic Charcot
    neuroarthropathy: a systematic review. In: 6th Annual International Symposium on
    the Diabetic Foot. Edited. Noordwijkerhout (The Netherlands), May 10–14, 2011.
25. Wilson M. Charcot foot osteoarthropathy in diabetes mellitus. Mil Med 1991;
    156(10):563–9.
26. Butalia S, Palda VA, Sargeant RJ, et al. Does this patient with diabetes have oste-
    omyelitis of the lower extremity? JAMA 2008;299(7):806–13.
27. Fleischer AE, Didyk AA, Woods JB, et al. Combined clinical and laboratory
    testing improves diagnostic accuracy for osteomyelitis in the diabetic foot.
    J Foot Ankle Surg 2009;48(1):39–46.
28. Crim B, Wukich DK. Osteomyelitis of the foot and ankle: diagnosis and treatment.
    J Diab Foot Complications 2009;1(2):26–35.
29. Shank CF, Feibel JB. Osteomyelitis in the diabetic foot: diagnosis and manage-
    ment. Foot Ankle Clin 2006;11(4):775–89.
30. Burns PR, Wukich DK. Surgical reconstruction of the Charcot rearfoot and ankle.
    Clin Podiatr Med Surg 2008;25(1):95–120, vii–viii.
31. Sammarco VJ. Superconstructs in the treatment of Charcot foot deformity: plantar
    plating, locked plating, and axial screw fixation. Foot Ankle Clin 2009;14(3):
    393–407.
32. Pinzur MS, Sage R, Stuck R, et al. A treatment algorithm for neuropathic (Charcot)
    midfoot deformity. Foot Ankle 1993;14(4):189–97.
33. Bevan WP, Tomlinson MP. Radiographic measures as a predictor of ulcer forma-
    tion in diabetic Charcot midfoot. Foot Ankle Int 2008;29(6):568–73.
34. Assal M, Stern R. Realignment and extended fusion with use of a medial column
    screw for midfoot deformities secondary to diabetic neuropathy. J Bone Joint
    Surg Am 2009;91(4):812–20.
35. Burns PR. Surgical management of malunions and nonunions of the diabetic
    neuropathic lower extremity. In: Zgonis T, editor. Surgical reconstruction of the

diabetic foot and ankle. Philadelphia: Lipincott Williams & Wilkins; 2009. p. 255–82.

36. Grant WP, Weinraub GM. Surgical reconstruction and stepwise approach to chronic Charcot neuroarthropathy. In: Zgonis T, editor. Surgical reconstruction of the diabetic foot and ankle. Philadelphia: Lippincott Williams & Wilkins; 2009. p. 230–40.

37. Disegi JA, Wyss H. Implant materials for fracture fixation: a clinical perspective. Orthopedics 1989;12(1):75–9.

38. Grant WP, Garcia-Lavin S, Sabo R. Beaming the columns for Charcot diabetic foot reconstruction: a retrospective analysis. J Foot Ankle Surg 2011;50(2):182–9.

39. Perren SM. The biomechanics and biology of internal fixation using plates and nails. Orthopedics 1989;12(1):21–34.

40. Pinzur M. Surgical versus accommodative treatment for Charcot arthropathy of the midfoot. Foot Ankle Int 2004;25(8):545–9.

41. Pinzur MS, Lio T, Posner M. Treatment of Eichenholtz stage I Charcot foot arthropathy with a weightbearing total contact cast. Foot Ankle Int 2006;27(5):324–9.

42. Brink DS, Eickmeier KM, Levitsky DR, et al. Subtalar and talonavicular joint dislocation as a presentation of diabetic neuropathic arthropathy with salvage by triple arthrodesis. J Foot Ankle Surg 1994;33(6):583–9.

Opening Wedge and Anatomic-Specific Plates in Foot and Ankle Applications

Andrew J. Kluesner, DPM, AACFAS[a],*, Jason B. Morris, DPM[b]

KEYWORDS

• Anatomic • Plate • Fixation • Wedge • Contoured • Locking

As surgeons continually push to improve techniques and outcomes, anatomic-specific and procedure-specific fixation options are becoming increasingly available. The unique size, shape, and function of the foot provide an ideal framework for the use of anatomic-specific plates. These distinctive plate characteristics range from anatomic contouring and screw placements to incorporated step-offs and wedges. By optimizing support, compression, and stabilization, patients may return to weight bearing and activity sooner, improving outcomes. This article discusses anatomic-specific plates and their use in forefoot and rearfoot surgical procedures.

ANATOMY

The musculoskeletal anatomy of the foot is comprised of unique structures and relationships that are distinctive from anywhere else in the human body. The foot is complex in its makeup and function. The joints and bones of the foot not only provide for motion but also provide the framework required for human bipedal gait. The intricate interplay of these structures allows the motion for propulsion but at the same time provides the stability to remain upright. During normal gait the foot must be able to withstand a force that is 1.2 times that of body weight with each step and 3 times that of the body weight while running.[1]

The shapes of the osseous structures that make up the human foot and ankle are unique. Foremost is the stable makeup of the medial longitudinal, lateral longitudinal, and transverse tarsal arches of the foot. Metatarsals are long bones each composed of unique articular shapes and surfaces. The bases of the metatarsal bones are mainly rectangular in appearance and articulate with the tarsal bones proximally, but with

[a] Department of Podiatric Medicine and Surgery, Christie Clinic, 1801 West Windsor Road, Champaign, IL 61822, USA
[b] University Foot and Ankle Institute, Santa Barbara, CA 93101, USA
* Corresponding author.
E-mail address: akluesner@christieclinic.com

Clin Podiatr Med Surg 28 (2011) 687–710
doi:10.1016/j.cpm.2011.06.005
0891-8422/11/$ – see front matter © 2011 Elsevier Inc. All rights reserved.

limited motion. These relationships are important in providing the shape, and therefore the stability, of the arches of the foot. The hind foot is comprised of the talus and calcaneus, with the articulation of these 2 bones allowing for the coupled triplanar motions of pronation and supination. The talus with its unique shape is almost completely covered in cartilage. This shape provides distinct articulations with the adjacent bones at the corresponding talo-calcaneal, tibial-talar, and talar-navicular joints; allowing for complex foot and ankle motion. The calcaneus provides stability and shape to the hind foot and has specialized osseous characteristics of a thin cortical outside shell and a soft cancellous filling.

These distinct anatomic features and complex interactions require special attention when addressing surgical correction of deformities and fractures. The importance of rigid internal fixation has been established as the standard in osseous surgery of the foot. However, applying this fixation to the anatomic constraints of the foot can be difficult. Historically, fixation devices that have been designed for other areas of the body have been used in the foot and altered as necessary to provide fixation. This procedure often requires additional operating room time, spent modifying and contouring traditional fixation. Bending plates to match the anatomy may not be ideal. Without proper contour, the plate does not allow for optimal compression in traditional fixation and may lead to suboptimal results. The goals to minimize morbidity, provide a stable mechanical alignment of the extremity and anatomic restoration of articular surfaces to maximize functional recovery have not changed, but advances in design and a better understanding of the biology of bone healing have provided new technology to better achieve these goals.

One of the major sources of morbidity associated with surgical procedures of the foot is the relatively prolonged course of nonweight bearing and the comorbidities that are often associated with this. Traditional fixation and plating systems have been designed to provide absolute stability by means of anatomic reduction and rigid internal fixation. The structural function of the bone is maintained in this situation and the major portion of the biomechanical loads remains with the bone.[2] The function of traditional plates and internal fixation in this instance is to provide compression, maintain reduction, and allow for primary bone healing. Traditional plating is typically not the main load-bearing element but more load-sharing. Because of this situation, weight bearing and loading of the surgery site are generally delayed until sufficient healing of bone has occurred, giving rise to a prolonged period of immobilization.[3] However, relative stability can be obtained by using an implant to bridge a fracture area while maintaining the anatomic axis, length, and rotation of the bone until consolidation has occurred. Healing is accomplished by callus or secondary bone healing. Locked plating technology is often utilized in this manner. Locked plates can be thought of as internal external fixators and are mainly load-bearing elements.[4] This technique produces stability and the potential to allow for earlier weight bearing, since the plate bears the load in the instance.

Numerous studies have supported the improved fixation behavior of locking plate technology compared with conventional plate fixation. Studies have shown favorable outcomes with locking plates, in particular when dealing with poor bone quality. Strength, number of cycles to failure, and displacement are all improved.[3–7] New plate designs now allow for locking screws to be placed at variable angles within the plate, facilitating better bone purchase, or better anatomic positioning of screws (**Fig. 1**).

Anatomic plates for the foot have been designed to account for the unique structure and also for some of the specific requirements needed to correct the various deformities of the foot. This situation has undoubtedly led to improved techniques and outcomes. These plates also aim to optimize fixation to achieve maximum stability or provide relative stability and possible earlier load bearing. Anatomic-shaped locking

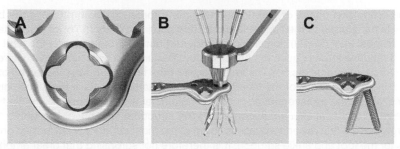

Fig. 1. (*A*) Variable angle locking hole design in plate. (*B*) Variable angle locking drill guide allows for locking screws to be placed within the locking hole up to 15° off axis. (*C*) Angled screw locked into plate. (*Courtesy of* Synthes Inc, West Chester, PA.)

plates are available that allow for compression application via proprietary forceps applied to guide pins placed within specialized slots in the plate before locking screw application (**Fig. 2**). This new technology aims at integrating properties from both of these principles by obtaining compression and providing relative stability and load-carrying properties, possibility decreasing the time required for immobilization.

FIRST RAY

The medial longitudinal arch serves as the chief load-bearing structure in the foot and is dependent on the kinematics of the first ray for optimal support during gait.[8-10] The first ray is a single foot segment consisting of the first metatarsal and the medial cuneiform. Pronation of the subtalar joint lowers the first ray to the ground in early stance and dissipates the shock of heel impact.[10] As body weight moves forward, the mechanics of supination stabilize the medial arch, preparing the foot as a rigid lever,

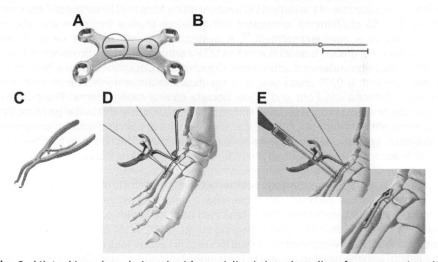

Fig. 2. (*A*) Locking plate designed with specialized slots that allow for compression. (*B*) Threaded compression pin used for temporary fixation between plate and bone. Ball on end of threaded portion of pin provides compression of plate to bone, and attachment point for compression forceps. (*C*) Compression forceps. (*D*) Compression forceps applied to pins, providing compression across fusion site before screw application. (*E*) Locked screws and plate maintain compression at arthrodesis site. (*Courtesy of* Synthes Inc, West Chester, PA.)

for the propulsive phase of gait. In normal gait, a force of about 120% of the body weight is transferred to the first metatarsal head and joint. Sixty to 75° of first metatarsophalangeal joint (MTPJ) dorsiflexion is required during propulsion. As the heel lifts, ground reactive forces cause the hallux to dorsiflex and the first metatarsal, via retrograde force, plantarflexes.[1,10] The importance of the first ray to the mechanics of the foot is, in part, because of the location of the metatarsocuneiform joint. This joint is located where the transverse and medial longitudinal arches intersect. The first ray, therefore, is a critical element in controlling the structural integrity of the foot.[9]

Surgery of the first ray encompasses some of the most commonly performed procedures for the foot and ankle surgeon. It is therefore not surprising that great emphasis has been devoted to the development of anatomic-specific plates to be used in the correction of foot and ankle disease about the first ray. With the significant force that is transferred to the first ray with ambulation many of these procedures require an extended period of immobilization to facilitate healing. Furthermore, the unique anatomy of the medial column and first ray make standard plate and screw designs difficult to use, requiring increased time to contour and maneuver. Anatomic-specific plates have been designed to take into account the anatomy, optimizing stability and decreasing operating room time needed to apply fixation.

FIRST METATARSAL PHALANGEAL ARTHRODESIS

An area that has gained significant attention is anatomic plate design for first MTPJ arthrodesis. First MTPJ arthrodesis has been shown to be an effective procedure for the treatment of many disorders affecting the joint, including end-stage degenerative joint disease or osteoarthritis (OA), joint destructive rheumatologic disorders, hallux rigidus, neuromuscular-associated hallux abductovalgus (HAV) deformities, HAV deformities with associated OA, and failed previous surgeries of the first MTPJ.[11–14] Arthrodesis of this joint has been shown to have high rates of union and patient satisfaction. The union rate of the patients in a recent study from the University of Pittsburgh was 94.8% (55 of 58 joints), consistent with previous studies that have also shown arthrodesis as a reliable treatment.[15] A systematic review of 1451 cases found a success rate of greater than 90% with first MTPJ arthrodesis.[16] In a prospective study of 49 patients who underwent arthrodesis, Goucher and Coughlin[17] noted a 96% satisfaction rate with a 92% union rate, and significant improvements in both pain and American Orthopaedic Foot and Ankle Society clinical rating scores. Preoperative and postoperative gait analysis have shown increased stability and better gait function in patients after arthrodesis.[18–20] Clinical improvement in pain and walking ease were also shown, with no changes in knee or hip kinetics found.[18] It has therefore become a widely accepted and performed procedure for the first metatarsal phalangeal joint.

McKeever,[21] who is credited for popularizing this procedure, has said "It is the fusion and its position that is important and not the method by which it is obtained." The importance of this cannot be overlooked, because a rigid malpositioned hallux inevitably leads to patient dissatisfaction. The established parameters for position include dorsiflexion of 10° to 15° from the weight-bearing surface, 10° to 15° of valgus in the transverse plane (usually referenced as parallel to a rectus second toe), and 0° of frontal plain angulation (with the nail bed parallel to the weight-bearing surface). Conical joint preparation techniques have allowed the surgeon to dial in correction and position the hallux with relative ease. Anatomic plating systems are designed to be precontoured to account for the position of the arthrodesis, allowing the plate to help position the arthrodesis and eliminate the bending and contouring that are required of a conventional straight plate (**Fig. 3**). The conical joint preparation technique in combination with

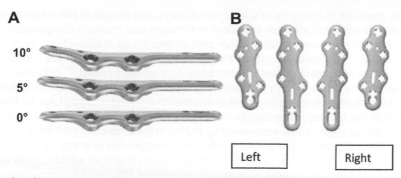

Fig. 3. (*A, B*) Precontoured first metatarsal phalangeal joint arthrodesis plates. (*Courtesy of* Synthes Inc, West Chester, PA.)

fixation by means of dorsal plate and crossed screw have shown significantly superior stability when compared with other methods.[22,23] Patients allowed immediate weight bearing have shown no significant difference in arthrodesis rates when compared with those kept nonweight bearing.[24] New locked plating designs aim to enhance stability and improve on already reliable outcomes (**Fig. 4**). By allowing the patient immediate postoperative weight bearing there may be a decrease in the morbidity.

FIRST METATARSAL OPENING WEDGE OSTEOTOMY

Trethowen in 1923[25] first described an opening wedge osteotomy of the proximal first metatarsal in the treatment of hallux valgus, but this was largely abandoned until

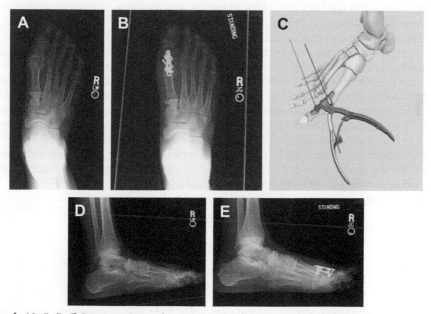

Fig 4 (*A, B, D, E*) Preoperative and postoperative first metatarsal phalangeal joint arthrodesis radiographs with the anatomic-specific locking compression plate. Patient was allowed immediate postoperative weight bearing in a walking cast boot. (*C*) Forceps provides compression across arthrodesis before placement of locking screws. ([*C*] *Courtesy of* Synthes Inc, West Chester, PA.)

recently because of concerns of stability and union. The benefit of this procedure lies in its ability to correct moderate to severe deformities and maintain and possibly even lengthen the first metatarsal. Many other procedures aimed at correcting moderate to severe hallux valgus deformities lead to shortening of the first metatarsal, with as little as 2 to 3 mm of shortening having adverse affects on the forefoot.[26] This situation is especially true in patients with a preexisting short first metatarsal. With the advent of improved fixation techniques and anatomic-specific opening wedge plates for the first metatarsal, this technique has regained acceptance (**Fig. 5**). The hallux valgus and first intermetatarsal angle can be addressed by dialing in the correction with this technique (**Fig. 6**). Recent studies have shown the first metatarsal base opening wedge osteotomy fixated with an anatomic-specific opening wedge plate is an effective method for correcting moderate to severe hallux valgus deformities and maintaining or even gaining length.[27–30] A success rate of more than 88% has been shown with this procedure, allowing patients early postoperative weight bearing.

FIRST METATARSAL CUNEIFORM ARTHRODESIS

Lapidus originally described an arthrodesis between the bases of the first and second metatarsals and the first intercuneiform joint to correct metatarsus primus varus in patients with hallux valgus.[25] The modified Lapidus procedure incorporates an isolated arthrodesis of the first metatarsal cuneiform joint. This procedure is typically reserved for moderate to severe deformities or those with relative instability or hypermobility of the first ray segment. This technique frequently involves fixation of the arthrodesis with 2 crossed screws. Patients are usually immobilized in a short leg cast nonweight bearing for 6 to 8 weeks. Nonunion (rates ranging from 5% to 15%) or malunion is the predominant cause of failure. The evolution of this procedure has involved improvement in fixation aimed at correcting these issues.[31] Numerous studies have reported successful outcomes with the modified Lapidus procedure, but uniformly report an extended course of nonweight bearing.[25] Interest is now focused on anatomic-specific plating designs to enhance arthrodesis rates of the first metatarsal cuneiform joint, provide further stability, and potentially allow for earlier weight bearing postoperatively. Multiple biomechanical cadaveric studies have shown the combination of an anatomic-specific medial locking plate combined with an adjunct compression screw to be a superior form of fixation than the traditional construct of 2 crossed screws.[32,33] Recent clinical studies have reported that the combination of anatomic-specific medial locking plate and compression screw allows for earlier postoperative weight bearing without any significant difference in complication rates compared with the traditional crossed screw techniques (**Fig. 7**).[34–36] However, further prospective studies are needed before making a final conclusion.

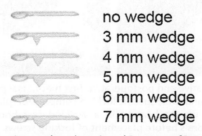

Fig. 5. First metatarsal opening wedge plate sizes. (*Courtesy of* Synthes Inc, West Chester, PA.)

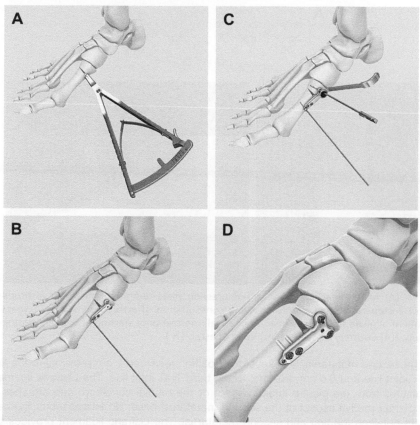

Fig. 6. (A) Distraction device with calibrated handle allows for osteotomy to be gradually opened medially to dial in correction desired. (B) Temporary fixation of plate with compression wire. (C) Variable angle drill guide for locking screws. (D) Anatomic-specific opening wedge first metatarsal locking plate. (*Courtesy of* Synthes Inc, West Chester, PA.)

LISFRANC ARTHRODESIS

Arthrodesis of the Lisfranc joint has been shown to be a successful procedure, with reliable outcomes for both the primary treatment of fracture/dislocations as well as posttraumatic reconstruction. Multiple studies have suggested primary arthrodesis as a treatment of Lisfranc joint injuries because of the high incidence of subjects undergoing open reduction with internal fixation (ORIF) eventually going on to require arthrodesis. If performed during the primary setting of injury, it negates a potential second surgery.[37,38] Reliable stability of the tarsal-metatarsal (TMT) joint has been shown with arthrodesis, and the need to remove hardware that is often required after ORIF is reduced. Arthrodesis continues to be the preferred treatment as a salvage procedure after primary ORIF, for delayed or missed Lisfranc complex injuries, and for severely comminuted intra-articular fractures of the TMT joints.[39–42] Furthermore, in patients who have failed conservative treatment with nontraumatic primary OA affecting the TMT joints, those with underlying systemic rheumatologic conditions, and those with neuropathic factures affecting these joints, arthrodesis remains an effective procedure.

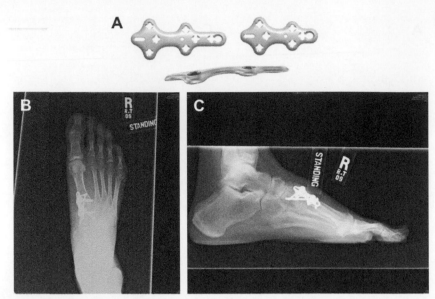

Fig. 7. (*A*) Anatomic-specific locking compression plate design for first TMT arthrodesis. (*B, C*) Postoperative radiographs showing consolidation of arthrodesis site at 7 weeks in a patient allowed full weight bearing in a walking cast boot starting at 3 weeks postoperatively. ([*A*] *Courtesy of* Synthes Inc, West Chester, PA.)

The second metatarsal is in keystone position recessed 1 cm proximal to the first TMT joint line and 0.5 cm proximal to the third TMT joint line. The Lisfranc ligament originates from the plantar lateral aspect of the medial cuneiform and attaches to the plantar medial aspect of the second metatarsal base. No interosseous ligament exists between the first and second metatarsal. The Lisfranc ligament provides the only soft tissue link between the first ray and the lesser metatarsals and is the major source of stability to the Lisfranc complex. Reconstruction of this area requires maintaining or restoring these anatomic relationships to provide stability of the midfoot. Motion of the TMT joints is variable, but it is generally accepted that the primary function of the first 3 TMT joints is stability and that of the fourth and fifth TMTs is motion. This theory is shown by the lateral columns giving roughly 3 times more motion than the first TMT.[10] This motion of the lateral column must be preserved to maintain normal function. On the other hand, arthrodesis of the first 3 TMT joints is generally acceptable to restore stability.

The unique anatomy of the Lisfranc joint complex can make fixation difficult. The first 3 rays have natural plantar declination from the cuneiform bone to the metatarsal base that continues down the metatarsal diaphysis to the head. Providing interfragmentary compression with screw fixation can prove challenging, especially with the narrow shafts of the second and third metatarsals. Exposure typically for these procedures can also lead to difficulty with interference of surrounding soft tissue and skin. Dorsal exposure of the medial 3 TMT joints is typically adequate with traditional skin incisions for these procedures. Plate fixation therefore provides an additional option to provide primary compression and stability of the arthrodesis sites, or as a secondary point of stability and fixation. First TMT plates are described in the previous section, but the natural declination of the second and third TMT make plate fixation with traditional minifragment plates difficult. Contouring of the plates is inevitable. Specific second and third TMT plates have now been designed to accommodate the unique anatomy of this area, providing compression and stability (**Fig. 8**). Although no specific studies have been published on the use of these plates, they do provide a fixation option for the foot and ankle surgeon.

CUBOID/NAVICULAR FRACTURES

Fractures of the midfoot tend to be less common than forefoot or rearfoot fractures. Most frequently, they present as stress fractures, avulsion fractures, or body fractures that are nondisplaced. This is in part because of the inherent stability of the midfoot through its structure and extensive network of ligaments. Generally, treatment consists of immobilization and rest. A lower percentage of these fractures are fracture dislocations, displaced, or comminuted fractures. Although less common, these types of injuries tend to require more aggressive treatment. This treatment may include closed reduction, ORIF, external fixation, or primary fusion. In these more severe fractures, compression and loss of structure can occur. Screw or Kirschner (K)-wire fixation has commonly been used for avulsion fractures or body fractures without comminution. When comminution is present or collapse of the bone has occurred, plate fixation is more useful. With the unique shape and structural importance of bones such as the navicular and cuboid, anatomic-specific plate designs are now available.

Navicular

The most common fractured midfoot bone is the navicular, which makes up 62% of these injuries.[43] Although there are many classification systems, fractures of the

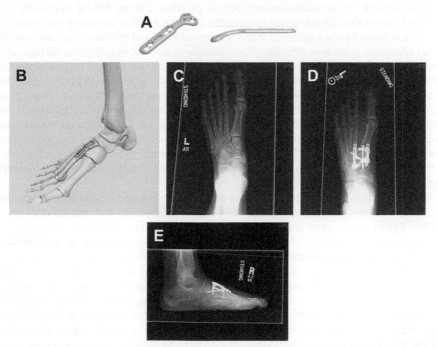

Fig. 8. (*A, B*) Anatomic-specific second and third TMT locking compression plate. (*C, D*) Preoperative and postoperative radiographs in patient with first and second TMT arthrodesis caused by missed Lisfranc injury. (*E*) The plate is contoured to account for the natural plantar declination at the second and third TMT joints. ([*A, B*] *Courtesy of* Synthes Inc, West Chester, PA.)

navicular can generally be divided into stress fractures, cortical avulsion fractures, tuberosity fractures, or body fractures. Cortical avulsion fractures typically occur from a twisting injury, leading to avulsion at ligamentous or capsular attachments. Mechanism of injury caused by forced pull of the posterior tibial tendon with the foot in an everted position results in the tuberosity fracture. Navicular body fractures occur after a high-energy crush injury, or adduction force. Because of this situation, articular surfaces are involved and bone structure can be lost. With the important position of the navicular in the midfoot, and its contribution to the talonavicular joint, anatomic reduction of these fractures is essential. It is in operative treatment of the navicular body fractures that the use of plates became an important method of fixation.

Early historical treatment of these fractures was either nonoperative or removal of the severely displaced fracture fragments.[43] In the 1950s, Bonavallet recognized the importance of the navicular in the foot structure and function, and advocated ORIF. He believed the poor anatomic reduction in conservative treatment resulted in the navicular losing its function as the cornerstone in midfoot stability.[44] Giannestras and Sammarco strengthened this idea and stated that closed reduction was of little value in displaced fractures of the navicular body.[43] Body fractures of the navicular continue to be considered among the most severe foot fractures because of their involvement with the talonavicular and naviculocuneiform joints. Current treatment recommendations reflect this situation, because all but the most minimally displaced fractures are treated with ORIF.[45]

Fracture patterns with large fragments can be repaired using just a single screw or multiple screws. When comminution occurs or when plantar lateral fragments are involved, screw fixation becomes more difficult. Plate fixation becomes more advantageous in these fracture patterns, but the shape and size of the navicular can present as an additional source of difficulty. The navicular is convex dorsally and distally, and concave plantarly and proximally. Standard plates such as the 1/3 tubular plate are difficult to contour along the dorsal surface. This plate provides less than adequate fixation and can become a source of irritation to the overlying soft tissue. The limited number of screw holes limits screw placement and therefore the usefulness of the plate in more complex fracture patterns. In some cases, secondary joint spanning bridge plate fixation or external fixation is needed to provide additional support lacking from the primary fixation.[45] These techniques provide increased stability in fractures with significant comminution or collapse, but a secondary procedure is usually required for hardware removal.

As anatomic plates have become more prevalent in foot and ankle surgery, specific navicular fracture plates have become available addressing the issues discussed earlier. These plates have characteristics that allow for successful use in an area of the foot where previous plates had limitations. The navicular plate is anatomically shaped, low profile, malleable and extends along the entire dorsal surface (**Fig. 9**). This plate limits soft tissue irritation and provides support to the medial, central, and lateral portions of the navicular if needed. An additional benefit is the variable angled locking screw design, which allows even more flexibility for fixation around a complex set of joints. For many plates, the screw holes are aligned in 2 rows, one proximal and one distal, to allow fixation at multiple points along the bone. Because of the thin profile, the plate can be cut and sized as needed.

The use of an anatomic navicular fracture plate is useful in displaced or mildly comminuted fractures. Although helpful in obtaining anatomic reduction and fixation, secondary fixation may be needed. Highly comminuted fractures or those with significant soft tissue trauma may require temporary external fixation or bridge plating to

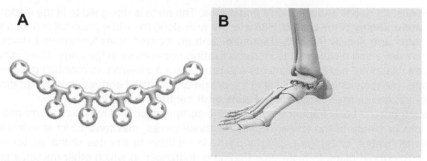

Fig. 9. (A, B) Anatomic-specific navicular fracture locking plate. (*Courtesy of* Synthes Inc, West Chester, PA.)

provide support and reduce collapse of the navicular. Simple fractures or nonunited stress fractures may require operative treatment, but tend to do well with compression and are typically fixated with screws or tension banding. When used appropriately, the plate can defend against dorsal tension and provides an additional fixation option of the navicular.

Cuboid

The cuboid is unique in its anatomy and is a wedge-shaped bone articulating with the calcaneus, lateral cuneiform, navicular, fourth metatarsal, and fifth metatarsal. Not only is its structure important in these joint articulations, but it also provides a groove for the peroneus longus and attachments for ligamentous structures. Fractures of the cuboid are mostly either avulsion fractures or compression fractures of the body. Avulsion fractures, which occur most often on the lateral aspect, are typically treated nonoperatively. Larger avulsion fractures or ones with significant displacement may require operative treatment. Compression fractures typically involve the entire body of the cuboid and because of the structural importance, are more serious. The mechanism of injury is characteristically a direct crush force or a fall with the foot in a plantarflexed position.[46] The name nutcracker fracture was given to cuboid fractures by Hermel and Gershon-Cohen.[43] This name refers to the fact that the cuboid is caught like a nut in a cracker with an abduction force trapped between the fourth and fifth metatarsals distally and the calcaneus proximally. The high force required to cause this type of fracture means it is typically associated with other injuries, including compartment syndrome and fractures of other midfoot bones.[44,46,47]

Displaced or compression fractures of the cuboid have had varying treatment protocols. In comminuted fractures with subluxation or dislocation some surgeons have advocated early midtarsal fusion.[48] As imaging and internal fixation techniques have improved, many now advocate ORIF.[43,49] This technique restores length to the lateral column and maintains the articulations to the adjacent bones. Historically, fractures of the cuboid have been repaired similar to navicular fractures. For minimally comminuted fractures, screws or wires are used. When significant comminution or compression is present, H-plates or 1/3 tubular plates are used as bridge plates to maintain lateral column integrity and length. The unique anatomy and characteristics of the cuboid provide the same challenges as the navicular with standard plating techniques available. Newer anatomic-specific cuboid fracture plates allow the surgeon to optimize fixation.

Similar to the navicular fracture plate the cuboid plate is a low-profile, malleable, variable angle locking plate. Titanium and stainless steel plates are available to fit the patient's needs and surgeon's preference. The plate is designed to fit the wedge-shaped anatomy of the cuboid, with a longer arm along the wider proximal aspect and a shorter arm distally (**Fig. 10**). There are centrally located holes for screws between the proximal and distal arms to increase fixation possibilities in the body. The design allows fixation of multiple fragments and provides a framework to maintain preinjury shape. The location of screws along the proximal and distal cortex allows restoration of length and permits placement of bone graft centrally if needed.

Many cuboid body fractures involve some compression and may be accompanied by loss of length in the lateral column. In these cases, maintenance of length with external fixation or bridge plating is useful in addition to the use of the anatomic-specific cuboid plate. In high-force trauma or instances in which other fractures are present, temporary fixation to maintain lateral column length may be used before ORIF of the cuboid, allowing for resolution of soft tissue injury before definitive fixation. The plate does provide an additional fixation option for the uniquely shaped cuboid and is another instrument in the surgeon's armamentarium for fixation of these fractures.

Calcaneal Fracture Plating

Treatment of calcaneal fractures, similar to the treatment of other foot and ankle conditions, has progressed as surgical techniques, instrumentation, imaging, and fixation devices have evolved. The 1 constant continues to be the complicated nature of these fractures. For this reason, some of the first anatomic-specific plates for the foot and ankle were calcaneal fracture plates, designed for the unique characteristics presented. These characteristics include the anatomy of the calcaneus itself as well as the unique fracture patterns associated with this bone. Calcaneal plates were increasingly used starting in the 1990s and have continued to develop. An understanding of the progression of calcaneal fracture treatment is paramount in understanding the development and use of calcaneal fracture plates. As the understanding and treatment protocol progressed, there was an increased necessity for fixation to advance as well.

Calcaneal fractures have been described since the times of Hippocrates and have presented difficulty for just as long. Described in 1708 by Petit and DeSault, the treatment of calcaneal fractures was initially rest until the fracture fragments had adequate time to consolidate. In 1908, Cotton and Wilson recommended closed reduction because of the difficulty of operative treatment.[50] The goal of their technique, which was typically performed using a mallet, reduced the lateral wall and width of the fractured calcaneus. Historically these techniques resulted in poor prognosis because the articular surfaces were involved in most cases and there was no attempt at reduction.

A   B

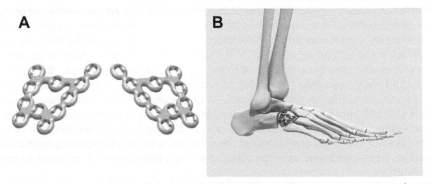

Fig. 10. (*A, B*) Anatomic-specific cuboid fracture locking plate. (*Courtesy of* Synthes Inc, West Chester, PA.)

Treatment can range from variations in closed reduction techniques to ORIF, pioneered by Leriche of France in the early 1920s. As early as 1938, Goff reviewed treatments of calcaneal fractures and listed 41 different operative technique.[50] Up to 75% of calcaneal fractures in adults are intra-articular, and the goal of treatment has been focused on reduction of the articular surfaces for better long-term results.[43]

In general, the advancement of surgical techniques has allowed for more accurate realignment of fracture fragments. By the 1960s, the treatment protocol that was generally accepted required meeting 2 goals. The first was restoration of the articular surfaces of both subtalar and calcaneal-cuboid joints. Second, bone morphology was to be restored, thus allowing for positional realignment of the articular surfaces.[51] Despite advancements in techniques and use of internal fixation, high complication rates were still associated with ORIF. Postoperative infection rates remained high and there were limitations in available fixation devices. Delayed subtalar or triple arthrodesis was commonly performed to treat the postoperative malalignment and arthritic sequelae.[52] This routine continued through the 1970s until French and Italian surgeons began treating more patients with ORIF using a lateral plate.[43,50,53]

As antibiotic prophylaxis became more common and fixation techniques improved, operative treatment outcomes improved as well. ORIF was increasingly used to allow more control over fracture fragment alignment. Historically, this was most beneficial for displaced, intra-articular fractures. By the early to mid 1980s, fixation was performed with screws and plates. These plates typically included 1/3 tubular plates or H-type plates. The use of both plates and screws allowed for better stabilization of multiple fracture patterns. Other benefits included reduction of the lateral wall, preventing triplanar motion of the calcaneal tuberosity, and resisting excessive bending forces. Although there were various surgical approaches, by the mid 1990s the most widely used became the extended lateral approach. This approach was most useful for displaced intra-articular fractures involving the posterior facet.[54] With the increased lateral exposure, plates became more common for buttressing the often comminuted and fragile bone. Additional support was gained and negated the used of additional bone graft in many cases.

The lateral extensile incision offers good exposure of the posterior facet and access to the lateral wall. This technique allows for an anatomic reduction of articular surfaces, as well as restoration of the height, width, and alignment of the calcaneus. This exposure does pose potential for complications including sural neuritis, peroneal tendinopathy, and wound complications, which is reported in up to 14% of cases using the extended lateral approach.[43,50] The incidence of deep infection is reported between 1.3% and 8%.[50] As these complications were noticed, the importance of minimizing surgeon-induced trauma and excessive stress to the area became evident. The goals of a specifically designed plate contoured to the lateral wall would help decrease excessive tension on the wound by maintaining a low profile, helping to establish and maintain reduction and, ideally, decrease surgical time.

HISTORICAL PLATE DESIGN

When first used for fractures of the calcaneus, the H-plate and 1/3 tubular plate were common. Other plates used included 2.7-mm dynamic compression plates, T-plates and L-plates. All of these plates had advantages over pins and screws by allowing buttressing along the lateral wall and increased stability. The H-plate was originally designed for use in anterior cervical fusions, but found use in foot and ankle surgery because of its unique ability to contour to the local anatomy. By allowing multiple screws in a relatively smaller area, it was used in fixation of arthrodesis and fractures.

The obvious disadvantages were that the shape, size, and screw placements were originally designed for a different anatomic area. With that factor in mind, these disadvantages were to be expected. It became evident that a plate designed and contoured for the calcaneus would be a great improvement over the current fixation options. By 1986, a calcaneal Y-plate began being used for ORIF of calcaneal fractures. The stem of the Y was placed along the anterior calcaneal neck and had 6 holes in case spanning of the calcaneal-cuboid joint was needed. One of the posterior arms ran to the posterior, superior calcaneus whereas the other was angulated toward the posterior calcaneal tubercle.[51] This new design provided a great improvement from the other available symmetrically designed plates. However, fracture plates continued to progress because there were still limitations in the new design. These first designs did not accommodate all fracture patterns encountered in severely comminuted fractures, and additional screws or plates were sometimes necessary (**Fig. 11**).

Sanders and colleagues in 1993[55] showed in their report of 120 displaced, intra-articular calcaneal fractures that anatomic restoration could be reliably obtained with ORIF. Postoperative computed tomography (CT) review revealed restoration in calcaneal height, length, and width as well as an anatomic reduction of articular surfaces. Bohler and Gissane angles were restored to within 5° of normal in all but 3 patients. These results were important because they showed an anatomic reduction of this challenging fracture could be performed and was reproducible. The information gained from this research and others during this time were critical in the next step of fracture fixation. With this information in hand, plate fixation used for calcaneal fractures continued to advance to accommodate fracture patterns and fixation needs for proper anatomic reduction.

CURRENT DESIGNS

By the mid 1990s the AO calcaneal plate had been developed. Calcaneal plates used today are the direct offspring of this design. They consist of properties that allow reduction and fixation of the major components of common fracture patterns. With large fragments, typically seen in extra-articular fractures, screws or smaller plates can still be used to obtain appropriate fracture reduction. Whether intra-articular or extra-articular, the current plates have the properties conducive to calcaneal fracture fixation. These properties are high strength, low profile, and shape design matching the calcaneal anatomy. Increased strength of the plate decreases the likelihood of plate fatigue and loss of fixation. Anatomic plate design allows for screw placement to accommodate the typical fracture patterns. A low profile allows for easy contouring and reduces peroneal irritation (**Fig. 12**).

For restoration of the posterior facet, many current plates have an angled portion of contour to be placed just beneath the articular surface of the posterior facet. This feature not only allows fixation after rebuilding and restoring the articular surface

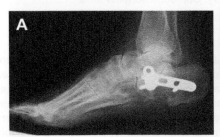
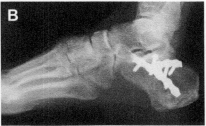

Fig. 11. Calcaneal fractures fixated with distal radial plate (*A*) and calcaneal Y plate (*B*).

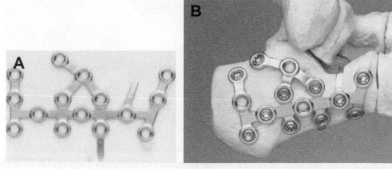

Fig. 12. Locking calcaneal plate (A). Plate contoured to saw bone model (B). (*Courtesy of* Synthes Inc, West Chester, PA.)

but also gives structural support to the unstable and once-depressed posterior facet. Whereas some plates have separate extensions beneath the facet, others have this feature as part of the body of the plate. Whichever plate is used, having this support along the posterior facet is critical in anatomic repair of intra-articular fracture patterns. Most plates also provide a locking design and may have variable angle placement of the locking screws. Because the calcaneus has a thin cortical shell and a soft cancellous interior, comminution is common. Locking plates provide increased stability because bicortical fixation of all screws is not likely to be obtained.

Another feature in modern calcaneal plate design is the strut support and additional screw placements along the anterior calcaneal neck and posterior calcaneal tubercle. Additional support and fixation are beneficial in fixation of any fracture type. The location of these plate features has come about secondary to critical steps in accurate anatomic reduction of calcaneal fractures. Varus malalignment of the calcaneal tuberosity is frequently seen in many calcaneal fracture patterns. The posterior portion of the calcaneal plate allows for fixation of the posterior-most components of the fracture, including the calcaneal tuberosity. As with the posterior facet portion of the plate, the anterior and posterior extensions typically have multiple holes for screw placement. Some of the plate designs allow for cutting or removing of unused holes along the periphery of the plate without compromising the structure of stability. Although the step-wise reduction may vary slightly, the reduction of the tubercle is important in restoring length, height, and rotational alignment of the calcaneus. The anterior process is often misaligned and in multiple fragments. Although variable, anterior extensions can have 2 or 3 holes to provide ample fixation in this area. By allowing stable fixation between the posterior and anterior calcaneus, the entire body of the calcaneus can be fixed to the sustentaculum tali, or constant fragment maintaining length, height, alignment, and articular reduction (**Fig. 13**).

Locking calcaneal plates have been shown to have greater stability during cyclic loading than plates without locking screws.[5,6] This situation provides increased stability and the potential for earlier weight bearing and mobilization, especially in significantly comminuted fractures. Variable angled locking plates allow more precise screw placement without sacrificing the locking capability. The locking screws may be placed at variable angles to allow for optimal bone purchase of the screws, and further anchoring to the constant fragment. Angled locking screws can also be used to fixate fragments that may not necessarily receive adequate fixation in the standard locking plate. Polyaxial locking plates have been shown to provide higher stability during

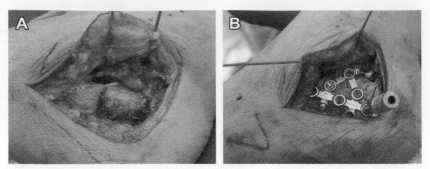

Fig. 13. Intraoperative calcaneal fracture before fixation (*A*) and after fixation (*B*) with locking calcaneal plate.

cyclic loading and limit posterior facet depression after load to failure compared with uniaxial locked designs (**Fig. 14**).[56]

Whether performing ORIF or primary subtalar joint arthrodesis for calcaneal fractures, the use of calcaneal fracture plating is the standard in operative treatment. It allows for stable fixation, restoration of calcaneal anatomy, and minimal soft tissue irritation. As techniques, medical technology, and treatment protocols have advanced, the quality of fixation has improved as well. Although calcaneal fracture plates have advanced, they are in no way a template for fixation. As Sanders and colleagues noted in their report of 120 calcaneal fractures, a learning curve is expected in calcaneal fracture repair. In type II or III Sanders CT classification patterns this learning curve may require up to 50 cases or 2 years' experience before consistent, predictable results can be expected. Each surgeon should select a plate design that works best with their technique, fracture pattern, and patient needs.

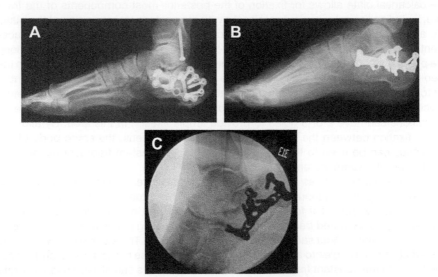

Fig. 14. Examples of current calcaneal fracture plate designs. DePuy perimeter plate (*A*). Synthes nonlocking calcaneal fracture plate (*B*). Stryker calcaneal fracture plate (*C*).

CALCANEAL OSTEOTOMIES/FUSION

Osteotomies of the calcaneus have been performed since Gleich described an osteotomy of the posterior calcaneus in the treatment of flatfoot deformity in 1893.[57] Many osteotomies have been described and used since; however, only a few have become commonplace in hindfoot corrective surgery. A medial displacement osteotomy of the posterior calcaneus was advocated by Koutsogiannus[57] in the early 1970s for correction of mobile flatfoot deformity. In 1975, Evans[58] described an osteotomy used to lengthen the lateral column in treatment of calcaneovalgus deformities.

For many rearfoot deformities, fusion of the subtalar joint or a triple arthrodesis has been a common form of surgical treatment. More recently, there has been a trend toward joint preservative methods because of the critical role they play in normal biomechanics of the foot during gait.[59] In particular, the treatment of flexible flatfoot deformities has seen the use of calcaneal osteotomies in conjunction with soft tissue procedures. Lateral column lengthening and posterior displacement osteotomy in particular are used routinely. Just as in other areas of the body, the frequent use of these procedures, anatomic characteristics, and fixation requirements have led to the development of specifically designed anatomic plates.

LATERAL COLUMN LENGTHENING

Procedures to lengthen the lateral column are performed by use of an osteotomy or distraction arthrodesis of the calcaneal cuboid joint. An osteotomy of the anterior portion of the calcaneus allows lengthening with the use of structural bone graft, typically tricortical, while keeping the calcaneal cuboid joint intact. This type of graft allows for structural support to maintain length and provides adequate cancellous bone for osteoconduction of the new bone incorporation. Osteoinductive properties typically rely on the source and preparation of graft, typically either allogenic or autogenic. When first described, Evans used 3 small cortical tibial grafts to maintain the obtained lateral length in his patients.[58] The osteotomy is made between 1 cm and 1.5 cm proximal to the calcaneocuboid joint.

When used in the appropriate patient, the Evans calcaneal osteotomy is beneficial in helping to correct flexible pes valgus deformity. In certain instances it has been shown to increase calcaneocuboid joint pressures and thus potentiate capsulitis or arthritic problems. Because of this situation, some surgeons advocate lateral column lengthening through calcaneal cuboid joint distraction arthrodesis.[60,61] This technique is performed through resection of the calcaneocuboid joint surfaces and use of structural bone graft to obtain length. In lateral column lengthening the oblique midtarsal joint axis becomes more perpendicularly oriented and results in decrease of forefoot abduction on the rearfoot. Deformity correction is obtained primarily within the transverse plane, but all 3 planes gain some correction.[62] Not only is forefoot abduction reduced, but it has been shown to plantarflex the first metatarsal and thus reduce subluxation of the talocalcaneal joint.[62] A review of 35 procedures by Mahan and McGlamry[63] showed an increase of calcaneal inclination angle, first metatarsal declination angle, and improvement in anteroposterior position of the talus.

The Evans osteotomy is typically performed using an oblique or slightly oblique incision just proximal to the calcaneocuboid joint. Once proper dissection is performed with freeing of the extensor digitorum brevis and retraction of the peroneal tendons, the anterior portion of the calcaneus should be visible and allow for completion of the osteotomy. As stated earlier, this procedure is typically performed 10 to 15 mm posterior to the calcaneocuboid joint. This is a through osteotomy because the axis of correctional rotation is near the center of the talar head.[62] Because of this situation a trapezoid wedge is preferred to obtain length. The lateral dimension of the graft is typically between 6 mm and 10 mm. For every 1 mm of lengthening obtained with graft placement along the lateral column, there is 1° of correction along the transverse plane.[64] Larger grafts can be used, but may cause increased pressures at the calcaneocuboid joint. Lateral column lengthening via calcaneal cuboid joint arthrodesis is performed through a more linear incision over the calcaneal cuboid joint. Graft size can generally be larger than in the Evans procedure because the removal of cartilaginous surfaces decreases some length and increase in adjacent joint pressure is minimal. Graft size is typically between 10 and 15 mm in lateral measurement.

Complications that are common in the Evans calcaneal osteotomy are structural collapse of graft, displacement of the graft, dorsal displacement of the anterior calcaneal portion, nonunion, peroneal tendon irritation, and sural neuritis. Nonunions have been reported as high as 20%.[65] In this same evaluation of calcaneal lengthening osteotomy, there was subluxation of the anterior calcaneus in 9.7% patients and displacement of the graft in 3.2% of patients. In calcaneocuboid joint distraction arthrodesis, there tends to be higher rates of nonunion and it is generally avoided in pediatric patients with open physis and growth potential.

Graft failure resulting in potential loss of correction, hardware failure, and chronic lateral pain continues to be the most common complication associated with both procedures. This complication is in part because the bone graft is the main structural support maintaining correction. Evans[58] originally described the procedure without fixation. This technique has continued, with many surgeons using no fixation or a single screw or K-wire. Plate and screw fixation is advocated when performing distraction arthrodesis of the lateral column because of the higher rates of nonunion and graft failure.[66,67] In a cadaveric study, Kimball and colleagues[67] showed a significantly higher stiffness and load to failure when using H-plate fixation compared with cross screws for distraction arthrodesis. The location of Evans osteotomy and calcaneocuboid joint distraction arthrodesis is separated by 10 to 15 mm. Although no data exist, it seems logical that when returning to weight bearing these 2 procedures undergo similar forces. Specific plate designs to accommodate the anatomy in this area, allowing the surgeon to dial in correction with the use of various sized wedges in the plate to maintain length, may help to combat some of the inherent complications associated with these procedures. More stability is obtained with the use of a fixation plate and may make it possible for earlier return to weight bearing.

PLATE DESIGN

Whether it is a combination of increased stability shown in H-plate constructs or the potential to bear weight earlier, the use of plate fixation has become more common with Evans calcaneal osteotomies. This situation has led to development and use of anatomic plate designs for these lateral column procedures. In the case of the anterior calcaneal osteotomy, wedge plates have shown potential in providing the stability seen in H-plate constructs with additional support of a wedge integrated within the plate. In the traditional technique, length is maintained by graft support. This feature can be the source of intraoperative and postoperative problems. If obtaining autologous structural graft, there is added comorbidity and increased surgical time. Once the graft is in place, it can be more difficult to obtain additional length if intraoperative examination reveals the correction to be inadequate. Furthermore, the on the table correction is often lost as normal bone resorption occurs over time as the graft incorporates. Using a wedge plate or wedge sizer, the surgeon can evaluate foot alignment and adjust the size of wedge as needed. This strategy eliminates the need for

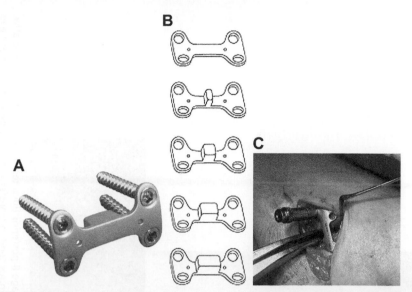

Fig. 15. Evans calcaneal osteotomy plate with wedge design (*A*). Examples of wedge sizes available (*B*). Intraoperative placement of the wedge plate after Evans calcaneal osteotomy (*C*). (*Courtesy of* Wright Medical Technology Inc, Memphis, TN.)

structural bone graft to maintain structural position and strength. The plates can be used to maintain length without the need of a structural bone graft, and potentially reduce complications such as anterior calcaneal dislocation or graft displacement.

Plates for Evans calcaneal lengthening osteotomy are designed with inward curvature of the superior and inferior portions to contour along the matching anterior calcaneal anatomy. Screw placement is aligned to allow inward convergence of 4 screws, 2 anterior and 2 posterior. Autograft or allograft bone can be used to fill in the wedged osteotomy site. Because of the higher nonunion rates associated with calcaneocuboid joint distraction arthrodesis, it is preferred to obtain length with bone graft. The length can then be maintained with the use of nonwedged plates, which may be available with the wedge plate set (**Fig. 15**).

There are limitations of the currently designed lateral column plates. The biggest limitation is in wedge size. Availability ranges from 2-mm wedges to 10-mm wedges. Many surgeons recommend the use of grafts up to 12 mm in lateral width.[67,68] These plates would not accommodate wedges of that size and would do better with a single structural graft with a nonwedged plate for fixation. Another limitation is in the biomechanics of obtaining the length only along the lateral most portion of the osteotomy. As discussed by Mosca,[68] the axis of correction is beneath the center of the talar head. Because of this, trapezoid bone grafts are used to allow lengthening along the entire osteotomy site. More length is obtained laterally, and less along the medial aspect of the anterior calcaneus. A wedge plate places the center of rotational correction along the medial calcaneal cortex. To obtain length similar to a trapezoid graft, one needs a smaller structural graft medially along with a wedge plate medially. There are no studies comparing patient outcome using a wedge plate versus using a structural bone graft (**Fig. 16**).

Although use of anatomic plating for lateral column lengthening does not necessarily decrease inherent complications associated with the anatomic location of the

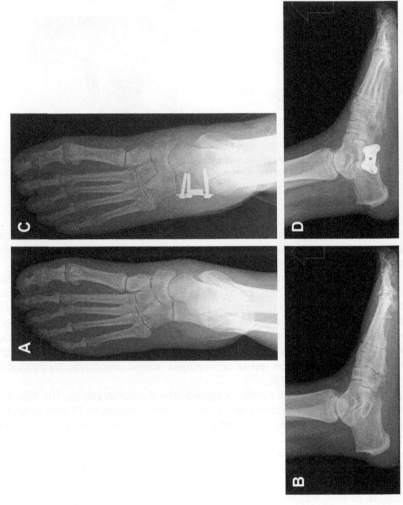

Fig. 16. Preoperative anteroposterior (AP) (*A*) and lateral (*B*) radiographs of a patient with stage II posterior tibial tendon dysfunction. Postoperative AP (*C*) and lateral (*D*) radiographs after Evans calcaneal osteotomy and flexor digitorum longus tendon transfer. Note the decrease in talar head uncovering and talus-first metatarsal angle after the procedure.

procedure, it may help limit other complications associated with graft displacement and loss of correction. The surgeon can select between a plate without a wedge or one with an inherent wedge design. Plate fixation has given surgeons the benefit of additional stability in lateral column procedures. This situation can allow earlier return to weight bearing and a quicker return to activity. As with other procedures, patient selection is important for optimal outcome. The lateral column plates offer an additional fixation option and, when used appropriately, show promise for use in these procedures.

SUMMARY

Fixation options for the foot continue to advance for many commonly performed procedures. As surgeons continue to improve technique an improvement in patient postoperative outcomes can be expected. The anatomic fit and design of recent plates along with the advances in locking screw technology and other intrinsic characteristics may allow the foot and ankle surgeon to achieve better outcomes and patient satisfaction.

REFERENCES

1. Nuber GW. Biomechanics of the foot and ankle during gait. Clin Podiatr Med Surg 1989;6(3):615–27.
2. Cordey J, Borgeaud M, Perren SM. Force transfer between the plate and the bone: relative importance of the bending stiffness of the screws friction between plate and bone. Injury 2000;31(Suppl 3):C21–8.
3. Perren SM. Evolution of the internal fixation of long bone fractures. The scientific basis of biological internal fixation: choosing a new balance between stability and biology. J Bone Joint Surg Br 2002;84(8):1093–110.
4. Seide K, Triebe J, Faschingbauer M, et al. Locked vs. unlocked plate osteosynthesis of the proximal humerus–a biomechanical study. Clin Biomech (Bristol, Avon) 2007;22(2):176–82.
5. Redfern DJ, Oliveira ML, Campbell JT, et al. A biomechanical comparison of locking and nonlocking plates for the fixation of calcaneal fractures. Foot Ankle Int 2006;27(3):196–201.
6. Richter M, Gosling T, Zech S, et al. A comparison of plates with and without locking screws in a calcaneal fracture model. Foot Ankle Int 2005;26(4):309–19.
7. Gardner MJ, Brophy RH, Campbell D, et al. The mechanical behavior of locking compression plates compared with dynamic compression plates in a cadaver radius model. J Orthop Trauma 2005;19(9):597–603.
8. Kotwick JE. Biomechanics of the foot and ankle. Clin Sports Med 1982;1(1): 19–34.
9. Mitchell LC, Ford KR, Minning S, et al. Medial foot loading on ankle and knee biomechanics. N Am J Sports Phys Ther 2008;3(3):133–40.
10. Valmassy RL. Clinical biomechanics of the lower extremities. St Louis (MO): Mosby; 1996. p. xviii, 510.
11. Lombardi CM, Silhanek AD, Connolly FG, et al. First metatarsophalangeal arthrodesis for treatment of hallux rigidus: a retrospective study. J Foot Ankle Surg 2001;40(3):137–43.
12. Yu GV, Gorby PQ. First metatarsophalangeal joint arthrodesis. Clin Podiatr Med Surg 2004;21(1):65–96.
13. Mann RA, Thompson FM. Arthrodesis of the first metatarsophalangeal joint for hallux valgus in rheumatoid arthritis. J Bone Joint Surg Am 1984;66(5):687–92.

14. Wu KK. First metatarsophalangeal fusion in the salvage of failed hallux abducto valgus operations. J Foot Ankle Surg 1994;33(4):383–95.
15. Sung W, Kluesner AJ, Irrgang J, et al. Radiographic outcomes following primary arthrodesis of the first metatarsophalangeal joint in hallux abductovalgus deformity. J Foot Ankle Surg 2010;49(5):446–51.
16. Coughlin MJ, Mann RA, Saltzman CL. Surgery of the foot and ankle. 8th edition. vol. 1. Philadelphia (PA): Mosby; 2006.
17. Goucher NR, Coughlin MJ. Hallux metatarsophalangeal joint arthrodesis using dome-shaped reamers and dorsal plate fixation: a prospective study. Foot Ankle Int 2006;27(11):869–76.
18. Brodsky JW, Baum BS, Pollo FE, et al. Prospective gait analysis in patients with first metatarsophalangeal joint arthrodesis for hallux rigidus. Foot Ankle Int 2007;28(2):162–5.
19. Brodsky JW, Passmore RN, Pollo FE, et al. Functional outcome of arthrodesis of the first metatarsophalangeal joint using parallel screw fixation. Foot Ankle Int 2005;26(2):140–6.
20. DeFrino PF, Brodsky JW, Pollo FE, et al. First metatarsophalangeal arthrodesis: a clinical, pedobarographic and gait analysis study. Foot Ankle Int 2002;23(6): 496–502.
21. McKeever DC. Arthrodesis of the first metatarsophalangeal joint for hallux valgus, hallux rigidus, and metatarsus primus varus. J Bone Joint Surg Am 1952;34(1): 129–34.
22. Buranosky DJ, Taylor DT, Sage RA, et al. First metatarsophalangeal joint arthrodesis: quantitative mechanical testing of six-hole dorsal plate versus crossed screw fixation in cadaveric specimens. J Foot Ankle Surg 2001;40(4):208–13.
23. Politi J, John H, Njus G, et al. First metatarsal-phalangeal joint arthrodesis: a biomechanical assessment of stability. Foot Ankle Int 2003;24(4):332–7.
24. Berlet GC, Hyer CF, Glover JP. A retrospective review of immediate weightbearing after first metatarsophalangeal joint arthrodesis. Foot Ankle Spec 2008;1(1):24–8.
25. Easley ME, Trnka HJ. Current concepts review: hallux valgus part II: operative treatment. Foot Ankle Int 2007;28(6):748–58.
26. Mann RA, Rudicel S, Graves SC. Repair of hallux valgus with a distal soft-tissue procedure and proximal metatarsal osteotomy. A long-term follow-up. J Bone Joint Surg Am 1992;74(1):124–9.
27. Wukich DK, Roussel AJ, Dial DM. Correction of metatarsus primus varus with an opening wedge plate: a review of 18 procedures. J Foot Ankle Surg 2009;48(4): 420–6.
28. Shurnas PS, Watson TS, Crislip TW. Proximal first metatarsal opening wedge osteotomy with a low profile plate. Foot Ankle Int 2009;30(9):865–72.
29. Randhawa S, Pepper D. Radiographic evaluation of hallux valgus treated with opening wedge osteotomy. Foot Ankle Int 2009;30(5):427–31.
30. Saragas NP. Proximal opening-wedge osteotomy of the first metatarsal for hallux valgus using a low profile plate. Foot Ankle Int 2009;30(10):976–80.
31. Cohen DA, Parks BG, Schon LC. Screw fixation compared to H-locking plate fixation for first metatarsocuneiform arthrodesis: a biomechanical study. Foot Ankle Int 2005;26(11):984–9.
32. Klos K, Gueorguiev B, Muckley T, et al. Stability of medial locking plate and compression screw versus two crossed screws for lapidus arthrodesis. Foot Ankle Int 2010;31(2):158–63.
33. Scranton PE, Coetzee JC, Carreira D. Arthrodesis of the first metatarsocuneiform joint: a comparative study of fixation methods. Foot Ankle Int 2009;30(4):341–5.

34. Saxena A, Nguyen A, Nelsen E. Lapidus bunionectomy: early evaluation of crossed lag screws versus locking plate with plantar lag screw. J Foot Ankle Surg 2009;48(2):170–9.
35. Basile P, Cook EA, Cook JJ. Immediate weight bearing following modified lapidus arthrodesis. J Foot Ankle Surg 2010;49(5):459–64.
36. Blitz NM, Lee T, Williams K, et al. Early weight bearing after modified lapidus arthodesis: a multicenter review of 80 cases. J Foot Ankle Surg 2010;49(4): 357–62.
37. Ly TV, Coetzee JC. Treatment of primarily ligamentous Lisfranc joint injuries: primary arthrodesis compared with open reduction and internal fixation. A prospective, randomized study. J Bone Joint Surg Am 2006;88(3):514–20.
38. Henning JA, Jones CB, Sietsema DL, et al. Open reduction internal fixation versus primary arthrodesis for lisfranc injuries: a prospective randomized study. Foot Ankle Int 2009;30(10):913–22.
39. Sangeorzan BJ, Veith RG, Hansen ST Jr. Salvage of Lisfranc's tarsometatarsal joint by arthrodesis. Foot Ankle 1990;10(4):193–200.
40. Mann RA, Prieskorn D, Sobel M. Mid-tarsal and tarsometatarsal arthrodesis for primary degenerative osteoarthrosis or osteoarthrosis after trauma. J Bone Joint Surg Am 1996;78(9):1376–85.
41. Komenda GA, Myerson MS, Biddinger KR. Results of arthrodesis of the tarsometatarsal joints after traumatic injury. J Bone Joint Surg Am 1996;78(11):1665–76.
42. Aronow MS. Treatment of the missed Lisfranc injury. Foot Ankle Clin 2006;11(1): 127–42, ix.
43. Rockwood CA, Green DP, Bucholz RW, et al. Rockwood and Green's fractures in adults, 6th edition, vol. 2. Philadelphia: Lippincott Williams & Wilkins; 2006. p. 2064–104.
44. Adelaar RS. Complications of forefoot and midfoot fractures. Clin Orthop Relat Res 2001;(391):26–32.
45. DiGiovanni CW. Fractures of the navicular. Foot Ankle Clin 2004;9(1):25–63.
46. Hunter JC, Sangeorzan BJ. A nutcracker fracture: cuboid fracture with an associated avulsion fracture of the tarsal navicular. AJR Am J Roentgenol 1996; 166(4):888.
47. Tountas AA. Occult fracture-subluxation of the midtarsal joint. Clin Orthop Relat Res 1989;(243):195–9.
48. Hermel MB, Gershon-Cohen J. The nutcracker fracture of the cuboid by indirect violence. Radiology 1953;60(6):850–4.
49. Sangeorzan BJ, Swiontkowski MF. Displaced fractures of the cuboid. J Bone Joint Surg Br 1990;72(3):376–8.
50. Rammelt S, Zwipp H. Calcaneus fractures: facts, controversies and recent developments. Injury 2004;35(5):443–61.
51. Letournel E. Open treatment of acute calcaneal fractures. Clin Orthop Relat Res 1993;(290):60–7.
52. James ET, Hunter GA. The dilemma of painful old os calcis fractures. Clin Orthop Relat Res 1983;(177):112–5.
53. Lanzetta A, Meani E. Operative indications in fractures of the calcaneus: problems of reduction and fixation. Ital J Orthop Traumatol 1978;4(1):31–5.
54. Benirschke SK, Sangeorzan BJ. Extensive intraarticular fractures of the foot. Surgical management of calcaneal fractures. Clin Orthop Relat Res 1993;(292):128–34.
55. Sanders R, Fortin P, DiPasquale T, et al. Operative treatment in 120 displaced intraarticular calcaneal fractures. Results using a prognostic computed tomography scan classification. Clin Orthop Relat Res 1993;(290):87–95.

56. Richter M, Droste P, Goesling T, et al. Polyaxially-locked plate screws increase stability of fracture fixation in an experimental model of calcaneal fracture. J Bone Joint Surg Br 2006;88(9):1257–63.
57. Koutsogiannis E. Treatment of mobile flat foot by displacement osteotomy of the calcaneus. J Bone Joint Surg Br 1971;53(1):96–100.
58. Evans D. Calcaneo-valgus deformity. J Bone Joint Surg Br 1975;57(3):270–8.
59. Pinney SJ, Lin SS. Current concept review: acquired adult flatfoot deformity. Foot Ankle Int 2006;27(1):66–75.
60. McCormack AP, Niki H, Kiser P, et al. Two reconstructive techniques for flatfoot deformity comparing contact characteristics of the hindfoot joints. Foot Ankle Int 1998;19(7):452–61.
61. Thomas RL, Wells BC, Garrison RL, et al. Preliminary results comparing two methods of lateral column lengthening. Foot Ankle Int 2001;22(2):107–19.
62. Sangeorzan BJ, Mosca V, Hansen ST Jr. Effect of calcaneal lengthening on relationships among the hindfoot, midfoot, and forefoot. Foot Ankle 1993;14(3):136–41.
63. Mahan KT, McGlamry ED. Evans calcaneal osteotomy for flexible pes valgus deformity. A preliminary study. Clin Podiatr Med Surg 1987;4(1):137–51.
64. Saxena A. Evans calcaneal osteotomy. J Foot Ankle Surg 2000;39(2):136–7.
65. Raines RA Jr, Brage ME. Evans osteotomy in the adult foot: an anatomic study of structures at risk. Foot Ankle Int 1998;19(11):743–7.
66. Deland JT, Otis JC, Lee KT, et al. Lateral column lengthening with calcaneocuboid fusion: range of motion in the triple joint complex. Foot Ankle Int 1995;16(11):729–33.
67. Kimball HL, Aronow MS, Sullivan RJ, et al. Biomechanical evaluation of calcaneocuboid distraction arthrodesis: a cadaver study of two different fixation methods. Foot Ankle Int 2000;21(10):845–8.
68. Mosca VS. Calcaneal lengthening for valgus deformity of the hindfoot. Results in children who had severe, symptomatic flatfoot and skewfoot. J Bone Joint Surg Am 1995;77(4):500–12.

Advancements in Percutaneous Fixation for Foot and Ankle Trauma

Ryan L. McMillen, DPM[a],*, Gary S. Gruen, MD[b]

KEYWORDS

• Percutaneous • Fixation • Foot and ankle
• Trauma • Minimally invasive

Operative fixation of foot and ankle trauma can be challenging. Often times, the soft tissue envelope can have extensive damage as a result of the fracture. In these cases, percutaneous fixation may be used. Soft tissue injury should always be respected by the surgeon. Understanding of both osseous and soft-tissue healing may help avoid common pitfalls with traditional operative fixation. Percutaneous fixation can benefit both soft tissue and osseous healing when used correctly. Many techniques have been described in the literature that may help to preserve blood supply, minimize soft tissue dissection, and restore a functional limb. This article reviews general guidelines for fracture and soft tissue management, osseous healing of fractures, and how certain techniques influence fracture healing. It also illustrates certain techniques for specific fracture reduction.

FRACTURE MANAGEMENT

The evolution of fracture care continues to advance and technology increases our understanding of soft-tissue injury, fracture healing, and how implants affect healing of both aspects. Before discussing percutaneous and minimal incision fracture repair, the evolution of managing soft tissue and fractures must be discussed. This philosophy is important to understand before percutaneous fixation can be used.

Soft tissue management is paramount in the setting of acute fractures. Respect for the soft tissue envelope will minimize complications following open reduction and

The authors received no external funding for this article.
[a] University of Pittsburgh Medical Center, 1400 Locust Street, Building B, Room 9520, Pittsburgh, PA 15219, USA
[b] University of Pittsburgh Medical Center, Division of Orthopaedic Traumatology, Kaufmann Medical Building, Suite 1010, 3471 Fifth Avenue, Pittsburgh, PA 15213, USA
* Corresponding author.
E mail address: mcmillenrl@upmc.edu

internal fixation (ORIF) or percutaneous fixation. Wound dehiscence, infection, and amputation are consequences of mismanagement or misunderstanding of the acute injury. Tscherne[1] developed a classification system for closed fracture grading recognizing that soft tissue injuries were often underestimated (**Table 1**). From his classification system, the Hanover fracture scale was developed to help grade traumatic injuries. This system is comprehensive and does not rely solely on the soft tissue or osseous injuries alone. It also includes the underlying soft tissue, vascularity, neurologic status, and contamination level of the injury; the time interval from injury to treatment; and the presence or absence of compartment syndrome.[1] This classification system is of practical use because it has been further updated and validated.[2] The personality of the soft tissue injury will affect the treatment and prognosis for healing. Fracture personality can be described by the type of force and the type of injury.

SOFT TISSUE INJURY

The pathophysiology of soft tissue injury is complex. The type of injury can help to determine the treatment required and the prognosis for healing.[3] The sequential healing process begins immediately after injury and is mediated by complex humoral and cellular mechanisms. This process can be subdivided into 3 phases. It is important to note that these are not distinct phases, but an overlap of the healing cascade. They include the inflammatory, proliferative, and reparative phases.

At the onset of injury, leukocytes interact excessively with the injured microvascular endothelium. A complex cascade of serotonin, adrenaline, and thromboxane-A is released causing vasoconstriction. Platelet-derived growth factor and transforming growth factor beta chemotactically attract macrophages, polymorphonuclear neutrophils, lymphocytes, and fibroblasts. Macrophages then respond to remove necrotic debris and bacteria.[4]

Kallikrein is released, which helps to improve vascular permeability by releasing bradykinin. Prostaglandins then stimulate the release of histamine from mast cells, which causes local tissue hyperemia. This action assists in the metabolic process of wound healing. Granulocytes and macrophages assist in the removal of cellular debris and microorganisms. These end products produced by macrophages and granulocytes mark the end of the inflammatory stage, which leads into the reparative phase.[5]

Fibroblasts and endothelial cells migrate toward the traumatized area and proliferate, which marks the beginning of the reparative phase. Collagen is then synthesized following the release of multiple cytokines. Fibronectins then facilitate collagen crosslinking by bonding type I collagen to alpha1 chains. Collagen cross-linking continues through a transition to the reparative phase. Proliferative endothelial cells form capillaries, which decreases water content. Type I collagen is then replaced by type III collagen, which results in fibrosis and scarring.[6,7]

Table 1		
Tscherne soft tissue injury classification		
Grade	**Description**	**Fracture Pattern**
C0	Little or no soft tissue injury	Mild
CI	Superficial abrasion	Mild to moderate
CII	Deep abrasion or local muscle contusion	Moderately severe
CIII	Extensive skin contusion, crushing, or muscle injury	Severe injury

FRACTURE HEALING

Clinical understanding of the surgical anatomy, characteristics of bone, and bone healing is also required when treating acute fractures. Bone healing is affected by many events and is impeded by the environment, the injury, and the surgeon. Healing occurs in 4 generally accepted stages: inflammation, soft callus formation, hard callus formation, and remodeling.[8]

Inflammation is a natural occurrence in all traumatic injuries. This process occurs quickly after the injury and is marked by hematoma formation, inflammatory exudation, and bone necrosis. Cytokines are released after platelet degranulation, which produces the inflammatory response of vasodilatation, hyperemia, polymorphonuclear neutrophils, and macrophages. Hematoma is gradually replaced by granulation tissue. Necrotic bone is removed by osteoclasts during this stage.

Secondary bone healing, also called soft callus formation or endochondral ossification, is defined as the time when fragments of bone are no longer freely moving. Shortening usually will not occur at this time; however, angulation and rotation are still possible. This process begins after the inflammatory period and is marked by progenitor cells stimulating osteoblast production and new bone. Capillary ingrowth is allowed to occur, which increases vascularity to the new callus bone. At the fracture gap, mesenchymal stem cells differentiate into fibroblasts and chondrocytes, resulting in extracellular matrix, which replaces the hematoma.

The conversion of soft callus to hard callus occurs over months. Intramembranous bone formation occurs as enchondral ossification at the fracture site. This formation continues from the periphery of the callus and continues toward the center of the fracture gap. The soft callus is then replaced by woven bone.

Primary or direct bone healing bypasses some of the indirect stages of bone healing. When interfragmentary compression is achieved, the fracture ends are in permanent apposition. Under absolute stability, minimal, if any, bone callus is formed. Haversian remodeling occurs within a week. Lamellar bone is produced, crossing fracture gaps. Cutting cones, osteoclasts that remove necrotic bone and osteoblasts, which follow the osteoclasts, bridge the fracture gap. Capillaries follow the osteoblasts to increase vascularity to the healing bone.

SOFT TISSUE MANAGEMENT

Soft tissue management is paramount in safely and effectively treating patients with lower-extremity trauma. Much of our clinical understanding of soft tissue management comes from literature concerning pilon fractures. Ruedi and Allgower[9] discussed open reduction and internal fixation of tibial plafond fractures in their classic article. Most of their patients had Arbeitsgemeinschaft für Osteosynthesefragen/Orthopaedic Trauma Association type A fractures (low-energy injuries/Tscherne type 1). As such, the investigators had good results with immediate open reduction and internal fixation.[10] Unfortunately, when this treatment was applied to injuries with higher-energy causes, increased soft tissue complications, including dehiscence and infection, resulted.[11] In the late 1990s, stabilization of fractures with external fixation and delayed ORIF became standard of care for acute osseous injuries with known or suspected soft tissue compromise.[12,13] This method has shown to decrease soft tissue complications. Although all foot and ankle injuries do not require temporizing external fixation, the basic tenets of soft tissue management should still be applied to all acute osseous injuries. Stabilization with a cast or splint in the immediate postinjury time frame is required. Patients should be instructed to ice and elevate the injured lower extremity. It is safe to make incisions when swelling has subsided and patients have a positive skin wrinkle test. In lower-energy injures, this could be the same day or as soon as 24 hours after the injury. In higher-energy injuries, it is prudent to wait until patients have a positive skin wrinkle test anywhere from 72 hours to 10 days.

Just as important as the decision to take patients to surgery is the decision about where to place surgical incisions. In percutaneous applications, large skin incisions are avoided; however, the basic tenets of preserving the blood supply to the soft tissues remains. Blood supply to the dermis comes from 2 primary sources: the direct vascular system, which is connected to the skin through the fascia and septa of muscles, and the musculocutaneous system's vascular blood supply.[14] There are 3 main types of vessels that supply the musculocutaneous system. Segmental arteries are branches of the aorta in terms of their perfusion pressure. They are usually located deep in the muscle that they are supplying. Perforating vessels pierce the muscle and septa and help to connect the segmental arteries to the cutaneous vessels. Cutaneous vessels either run parallel to the dermis or course perpendicular to the skin surface. These cutaneous vessels form plexus, which are known as angiosomes. An angiosome is defined as a 3-dimensional composite unit of skin and the underlying deep tissue that is supplied by a single source artery.[15] The angiosomes of the lower extremity have been well mapped out and are exceptionally important when planning skin incisions in trauma surgery.[16] When closing incisions, it is generally accepted practice to minimize the use of forceps at the dermal layer to minimize compromise of the vascularity of the dermis. Electrocautery should be avoided at this level, and wound healing depends on the maintained microcirculation and viable tissue at the wound edges.

INDICATIONS

Indications for percutaneous fixation include, but are not limited to, complicated soft tissue environment, areas of known hypovascularity, minimal or no displacement of fracture fragments, and well-reduced fractures with closed reduction techniques. Regarding the foot and ankle, the complicated soft tissue environment can include high-energy pilon fractures, calcaneal fractures, or any fracture resulting in fracture blisters. Areas of hypovascularity include the distal tibia, the fifth metatarsal base, and the central portion of the navicular.[17,18]

EVOLUTION

The evolution of implant technology has contributed greatly to the application of percutaneous or minimally invasive techniques. These techniques involve little, if any, soft tissue or periosteal stripping, which results in increased blood supply to the surrounding fracture and presumably increased healing potential.[19] Locked plate technology allows the land of the screw to insert directly into the plate, locking in place. The plate is rigid, even if not directly compressed to the bone. With practice, this can allow for indirect reduction techniques of the fracture and percutaneous application of the plate and screws. This technique is called minimally invasive plate osteosynthesis or MIPO.[20] The concept of MIPO allows for percutaneous placement of a plate and screws, which minimally disrupts blood supply. The fracture hematoma is left in place. This practice helps to increase callus formation and allows for a more successful, uneventful healing environment.[21,22]

There were many advances to plate and screw technology that resulted in the MIPO technique and locking compression plates (LCP). The first advancement was the dynamic compression plate (DCP). Conventional plating methods require friction of the plate on the bone to achieve stability. This friction can drastically reduce periosteal blood supply.[23] Consequently, the limited-contact DCP was introduced to decrease the actual contact area of the plate to the bone, which is accomplished by having recessed areas on the undersurface of the plate. The plate still uses friction to achieve its stability; however, the blood supply interruption is drastically reduced.[24]

The next advancement was the less invasive stabilization system. This technology allows for the land to screw directly into the plate, locking it in place, which reduces the compressive forces on bone but also allows for the plate to be placed off of the bone so that the blood supply is not affected.[25,26] The disadvantage of using a locking plate system is the need to place a screw perpendicular to the plate. Locking and non-locking holes were then incorporated into the plate, forming combination or combi holes. These holes allowed for a locking screw to be inserted when increased rigidity was required or a nonlocking screw when the surgeon needed to place a screw at any angle other than 90° to the plate.[27]

With improvement, the LCP has been redesigned to accept many screw types. These types include standard cortical screws, standard cancellous screws, locking screws, self-drilling screws, and self-tapping screws. Conventional screws allow for insertion at an angle less than 90° to the plate. Locking screws should be inserted at an angle of 90° to the plate.[28] Appropriate application of the screw is based on the personality of the fracture as well as the desired application to achieve fracture union. First and foremost, screws should be placed interosseous and extra-articular. Secondly, they should not interfere with each other. The quality of the patients' bone can determine the type of screw that will be needed. Working length of cortical bone is an important concept to understand. The larger the width of the bone, the better purchase a bicortical nonlocking screw will have. This larger width allows for more surface area and, by design, more threads to purchase strong cortical bone. Locking screws need not be placed bicortical; however, doing so can also help to increase rotational stability.[24]

PERCUTANEOUS FIXATION
Central Metatarsals

Central metatarsal fractures are defined as fractures of the second, third, and fourth metatarsals. These fractures often occur distally at the metatarsal heads. Indications for open reduction and internal fixation include greater than 4 mm of displacement in any plane, greater than 10° of angulation, and multiple metatarsal fractures.[29] These guidelines are not always as rigid, particularly when there is sagittal plane deformity, but most will accept less than the 4 mm of displacement or 10° of angulation. Percu-taneous fixation of distal metatarsal fractures has been described in 2 ways. The first is the buttress concept. The fifth metatarsal head is used to stabilize the fractured central metatarsals. The k-wire is drilled through the fifth metatarsal head and into the reduced fractured central rays. This procedure allows for both stabilization and anatomic alignment without damaging the articular surface of the metatarsal head.[30] The second technique involves retrograde intramedullary percutaneous pinning of each individual central metatarsal fracture. This concept is considered the gold stan-dard for central metatarsal fractures.[31] This technique can be difficult because of the ligamentous and muscular attachments surrounding the metatarsal head. For this reason, the use of bone-holding forceps has been used to help stabilize and reduce the metatarsal head while the k-wire is being inserted in a retrograde fashion (**Fig. 1**).[32]

Fifth Metatarsal

Fractures of the fifth metatarsal are classified as distal or proximal. Most distal meta-tarsal fractures can be treated conservatively.[31] Proximal metatarsal fractures, classi-cally, the Jones fracture, are now classified into 3 distinct zones. These zones include

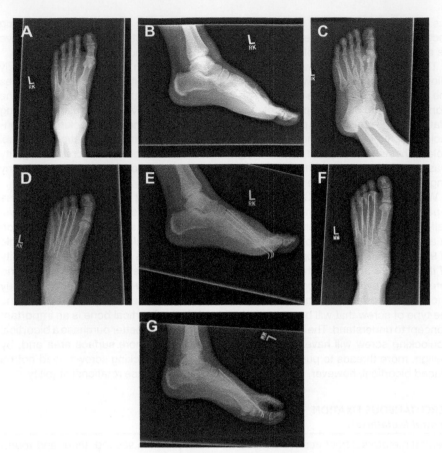

Fig. 1. (*A* and *B*) Initial injury radiograph. (*C, D, E*) Immediate post operative radiographs. (*F* and *G*) 8 week post operative radiographs.

avulsion fractures that occur from the pull of the peroneus brevis or lateral band of the plantar fascia.[33] Classifying proximal fifth metatarsal fractures helps to determine the appropriate treatment. Although many classifications systems exist for fifth metatarsal fractures, the zone concept has been used more recently to determine surgical intervention.[34] Most investigators support conservative treatment of zone 1 injures, which is an avulsion fracture of the fifth metatarsal tuberosity. Although many treatment options have been described, intramedullary fixation of zone 2 and 3 injures is the current standard.[35] Percutaneous insertion has been described for insertion of intramedullary screw fixation of fifth metatarsal fractures.[36] Although this technique helps to maintain the tenuous blood supply to the proximal fifth metatarsal, it is not without consequence.[17] Other investigators have suggested that a small mini-open incision should be used to preserve the sural nerve.[37] ORIF of fifth metatarsal fractures tends to achieve union faster than nonoperative treatment and is suggested for athletes or for patients who do not want to experience long periods of non–weight bearing (**Fig. 2**).[38]

Lisfranc Fractures

Lisfranc fracture/dislocation is a complicated injury. The anatomy of the Lisfranc joint and the associated injury patterns can make anatomic reduction difficult. Current

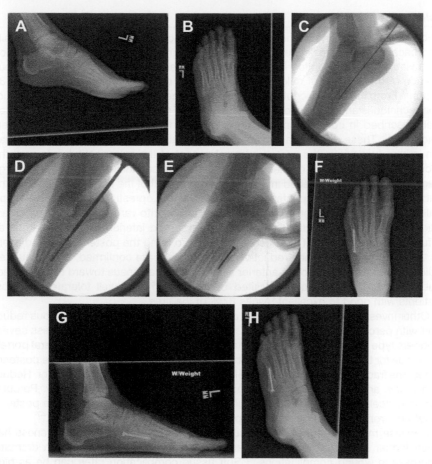

Fig. 2. (*A* and *B*) Initial injury radiograph. (*C, D, E*) Intra operative fluoroscopy of percutaneous fixation. (*F, G, H*) 6 Month post operative radiograph showing complete consolidation of jones fracture.

practice is open reduction and internal fixation or primary arthrodesis of the medial 3 rays.[39,40] However, there are investigators who have advocated closed reduction and percutaneous fixation of the acute Lisfranc injury. One large retrospective review article demonstrated that anatomic or near anatomic reduction can result in a satisfactory result. Forty-two patients were followed for an average of 58 months. Indications for closed reduction included closed injuries reducible by manipulative maneuvers, regardless of the magnitude of the dislocation and deformity. At final follow-up, the average American Orthopaedic Foot and Ankle Score was 81. The investigators found no significant difference in patients with anatomic reduction compared with near anatomic reduction. However, there was statistical significance in patients who had primary ligamentous injures compared with those who had osseo-ligamentous injures. In this study, those with ligamentous injuries fared worse.[41] Although this article does show promise for closed reduction and percutaneous fixation with cannulated screws for Lisfranc injuries, it should be noted that, In a review article of Lisfranc injuries, this was the only percutaneous fixation article written from 1985 to 2010 in the English language.[42]

Calcaneal Fractures

Because of the high incidence of wound complications with the lateral expansile approach for ORIF of calcaneal fracture,[43] percutaneous fixation has gained traction as a viable treatment option for intraarticular calcaneal fractures. The percutaneous fixation of these types of calcaneal fractures has been described for more than 30 years.[44] From the first description, much advancement has been made, both in reduction techniques and the fixation used. The classic Essex-Lopresti maneuver has been well described in conjunction with percutaneous fixation of intraarticular calcaneal fractures.[45] These patients are placed in a lateral decubitus position. A Steinman pin is introduced from the posterior lateral aspect of the calcaneal tuber toward the most inferior aspect of the displaced posterior facet. A cannulated guidewire for a large fragment screw is then placed into the posterior aspect of the calcaneus aimed at the subchondral bone of the posterior facet. The Essex-Lopresti maneuver is then typically performed in 3 motions: First, the foot is forced into varus to unlock the primary fracture. Second, the midfoot and first pin are forced inferior using the thumbs as a fulcrum. Finally, the foot is forced into valgus to bring the posterior facet adjacent to the sustentaculum. When reduction and alignment are confirmed, the cannulated guidewire is advanced into the anterior aspect of the calcaneus toward the calcaneocuboid joint. This technique, revisited by Tornetta,[45] was well tolerated by most patients with good to excellent results 87% of the time.

Other investigators have advocated arthroscopically assisted percutaneous reduction with percutaneous screw fixation. This technique has been used for less severe Sanders type IIA and IIB fractures.[46] Standard anterolateral and posterolateral portals are made for the arthroscope. A small incision is then made at the level of the posterior facet. The fracture fragments are then lifted and reduced with a sharp elevator. Reduction in this article was judged with image intensification and arthroscopy. Percutaneous cancellous screws were then placed as rafting screws beneath the posterior facet and from lateral to medial to help reduce the width of the calcaneus.[47]

Because more surgeons have pursued these techniques, their effectiveness has been further studied. The major advantage to percutaneous fixation is a dramatic decrease in wound complications.[48] Soft tissue complication rates can be as high as 14% to 20%, with up to 20% of patients needing a return trip to the operating room for soft tissue compromise.[49,50] Others have shown that a 2-layer approach to closure of the lateral expansile incision can reduce soft tissue complications.[51]

However, percutaneous reduction and fixation of calcaneal fractures is not without its own set of complications. A retrospective review of cases at least 1 year out of surgery showed altered gait biomechanics. The investigators found significant differences in weight distribution, total contact time, and the maximum pressure under the first metatarsal after a median follow-up of 18 months.[52] Still, other investigators have found subsidence of the posterior facet with percutaneous screw fixation.[45] However, the reduction maneuvers are complex and there are pitfalls to percutaneous reduction and fixation of calcaneal fractures. The use in less severe fractures has been shown to help reduce soft tissue complications and the need for arthrodesis of the subtalar joint at long-term follow-up (**Fig. 3**).[47]

Talus Fractures

Talar fractures are complicated injuries that usually occur through a high-energy mechanism. Previous orthopaedic practice was to treat talar neck fractures as surgical emergencies.[53] However, recent studies have shown no increase in avascular necrosis with increased time to operative intervention.[54] Avascular necrosis is of great concern

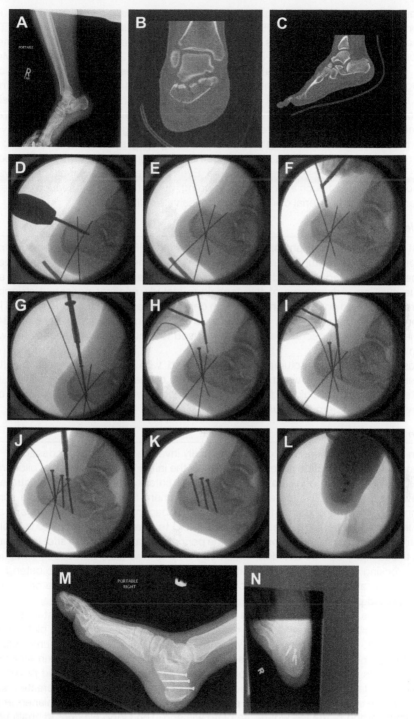

Fig. 3. (*A*) Initial injury radiograph. (*B* and *C*) CT Images of fracture pattern. (*D–L*) Intra operative steps for reduction of fracture and internal fixation. (*M* and *N*) 3 month post operative radiographs.

because of the tenuous blood supply to the talus. Avascular necrosis was previously reported as high as 90% to 100% with high-energy injuries and displacement.[55] The primary blood supply to the talus is the artery to the tarsal canal.[56] Current recommendations for open reduction and internal fixation include a 2-incision approach. Most talar neck fractures have medial-sided comminution. Thus, the reduction is difficult to judge based solely on the anteromedial incision. Varus malalignment is common with malreduction of the medial talar neck. For this reason, an anterolateral incision is recommended to help judge the reduction.[57] Percutaneous fixation is not often recommended for talar neck fractures. However, some investigators have reported favorable results.[58,59] In cases where a computed tomography scan has shown little to no comminution and there is little to no displacement (Hawkins type I and II), percutaneous fixation of talar fractures can be entertained. Even so, the surgeon should have a valid reason for the use of such a technique, including, but not limited to, tobacco usage by patients, peripheral arterial disease, and excessive swelling.

Ankle Fractures

Most ankle fractures can and should be treated with ORIF. However, certain subtypes of fibular and tibia fractures can be treated with percutaneous fixation.[60,61] Indications for percutaneous reduction include transverse Weber B and C fibula fractures with soft tissue swelling. Advantages of this technique include minimal periosteal stripping; decreased wound complications, including dehiscence and infection; and minimal irritation to the peroneal tendons. This technique provided good to excellent results 84% of the time.[61,62] This technique can also be used for fibula fractures associated with pilon injuries.

Posterior malleolar fractures are often treated with percutaneous fixation. It is generally accepted that when greater than 25% of the ankle joint is involved, the posterior malleolus should be fixed.[63] Many surgeons will perform the reduction and screw placement percutaneously.

Pilon Fractures

Pilon fractures have been treated with minimally invasive techniques for decades.[64,65] Spanning external fixation is now mandatory in the initial treatment stage of pilon fractures.[12,13] Many surgeons have advocated percutaneous placement of strategic screws with external fixation as a definitive treatment method. As plate and screw technology evolved, external fixation with MIPO became the current standard and can increase functional results.[66] Using the MIPO technique is advantageous in pilon fractures for many reasons. It preserves the periosteum at the fracture site; the zone of soft tissue injury can be avoided, which can help to decrease soft tissue complications; locking plates promote endosteal bone healing by preserving the osteogenic fracture hematoma; and the diaphyseal fracture can be bridged with the percutaneously placed plate.[67,68]

Techniques have been developed for percutaneous plating of the distal tibia that are reproducible and provide good results. General considerations are plate length and contour. There are now many commercially available precontoured plates. Length can be established with the use of fluoroscopy before any skin incisions. An incision is then made at the tip of the medial malleolus and extended proximally so that the plate can be easily passed. A Cobb elevator is then used to create a submuscular, extraperiosteal tunnel for plate passage. An incision is then placed at the proximal portion of the leg where the plate will end. The Cobb elevator is again used to make a tunnel for the plate from proximal to distal. A stout suture is wrapped around the most proximal hole of the plate. Pituitary forceps are placed from the proximal incision to the distal medial incision. The suture is grasped with the forceps and the plate is passed retrograde along the tibia.[68] This technique can be accompanied by mini-open or percutaneous reduction of any intraarticular fractures (**Figs. 4** and **5**).

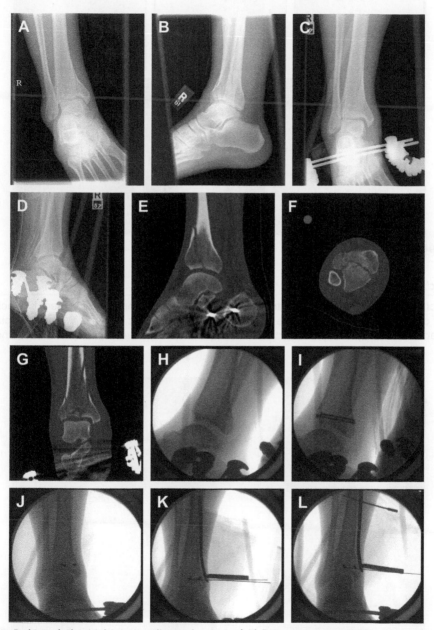

Fig. 4. (*A* and *B*) Initial injury radiographs. (*C* and *D*) Following External Fixation Application. (*E, F* and *G*) CT Images of fracture pattern. (*H–P*) Intra-operative steps for percutaneous placement of plate and screws. (*Q* and *R*) 4 Month post operative radiographs showing complete healing of fracture pattern.

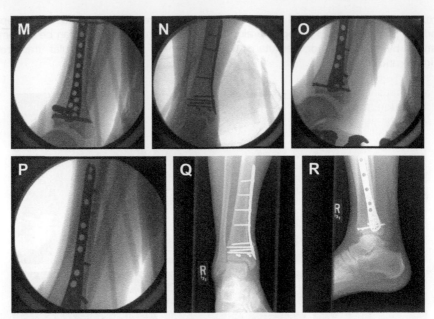

Fig. 4. (*continued*)

Achilles Tendon

Achilles tendon rupture can be treated operatively and nonoperatively. There is a lack of consensus in the literature as to which method is best for patients. Wound complications are the primary complication with open repair. However, rerupture rates and

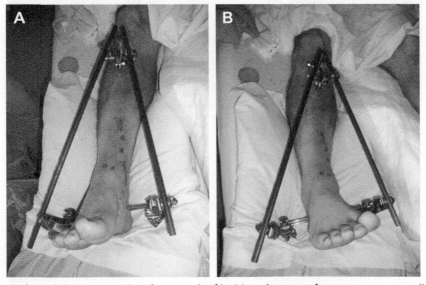

Fig. 5. (*A* and *B*) Post operative photograph of incision placement for percutaneous medical plate following pilon fracture.

lack of strength are higher in patients treated nonoperatively.[69] As such, many investigators have advocated percutaneous repair.[70,71] Ma and Griffith[72] were the first to report their technique of percutaneous repair. Many investigators have since attempted this technique. It was originally thought that the percutaneous repair gave the surgeon the best of both worlds in that there were little to no reruptures and no wound complications. However, studies have subsequently shown injury to the sural nerve and rerupture rates to be as high as 13%.[73,74] Although there seems to be no consensus as to which treatment method is best, the percutaneous technique may be an option.

SUMMARY

Percutaneous fixation in foot and ankle trauma is a challenge. There is a decreased soft tissue envelope compared with other areas of the body. Blood supply can be easily compromised with approaches and fixation. Soft tissue injury is of primary concern. Through the use of indirect reduction techniques, percutaneous screw and plate placement, and external fixation, the surgeon can help to minimize soft tissue damage and restore function to the injured lower extremity.

REFERENCES

1. Tscherne H, Oestern HJ. A new classification of soft-tissue damage in open and closed fractures (author's transl). Unfallheilkunde 1982;85:111–5 [in German].
2. Brumback RJ, Jones AL. Interobserver agreement in the classification of open fractures of the tibia. The results of a survey of two hundred and forty-five orthopaedic surgeons. J Bone Joint Surg Am 1994;76:1162–6.
3. Levin S. Personality of soft tissue injury. Tech Orthop 1995;10:65–73.
4. Steenfos HH. Growth factors and wound healing. Scand J Plast Reconstr Surg Hand Surg 1994;28:95–105.
5. van der Vusse GJ, van Bilsen M, Reneman RS. Ischemia and reperfusion induced alterations in membrane phospholipids: an overview. Ann N Y Acad Sci 1994;723: 1–14.
6. Schmid P, Itin P, Cherry G, et al. Enhanced expression of transforming growth factor-beta type I and type II receptors in wound granulation tissue and hypertrophic scar. Am J Pathol 1998;152:485–93.
7. Wu L, Siddiqui A, Morris DE, et al. Transforming growth factor beta 3 (TGF beta 3) accelerates wound healing without alteration of scar prominence. Histologic and competitive reverse-transcription-polymerase chain reaction studies. Arch Surg 1997;132:753–60.
8. Claes L, Heitemeyer U, Krischak G, et al. Fixation technique influences osteogenesis of comminuted fractures. Clin Orthop Relat Res 1999;(365):221–9.
9. Ruedi T, Allgower M. Late results after operative treatment of fractures of the distal tibia (pilon tibial fractures) (author's transl). Unfallheilkunde 1978;81: 319–23 [in German].
10. Ruedi TP, Allgower M. The operative treatment of intra-articular fractures of the lower end of the tibia. Clin Orthop Relat Res 1979;(138):105–10.
11. Dillin L, Slabaugh P. Delayed wound healing, infection, and nonunion following open reduction and internal fixation of tibial plafond fractures. J Trauma 1986; 26:1116–9.
12. Sirkin M, Sanders R, DiPasquale T, et al. A staged protocol for soft tissue management in the treatment of complex pilon fractures. J Orthop Trauma 1999;13:78–84.

13. Patterson MJ, Cole JD. Two-staged delayed open reduction and internal fixation of severe pilon fractures. J Orthop Trauma 1999;13:85–91.
14. Daniel RK, Williams HB. The free transfer of skin flaps by microvascular anastomoses. An experimental study and a reappraisal. Plast Reconstr Surg 1973;52: 16–31.
15. Taylor GI, Palmer JH. The vascular territories (angiosomes) of the body: experimental study and clinical applications. Br J Plast Surg 1987;40:113–41.
16. Attinger C, Cooper P, Blume P, et al. The safest surgical incisions and amputations applying the angiosome principles and using the Doppler to assess the arterial-arterial connections of the foot and ankle. Foot Ankle Clin 2001;6:745–99.
17. Smith JW, Arnoczky SP, Hersh A. The intraosseous blood supply of the fifth metatarsal: implications for proximal fracture healing. Foot Ankle 1992;13:143–52.
18. Waugh W. The ossification and vascularisation of the tarsal navicular and their relation to Kohler's disease. J Bone Joint Surg Br 1958;40:765–77.
19. Ozkaya U, Parmaksizoglu AS, Gul M, et al. Minimally invasive treatment of distal tibial fractures with locking and non-locking plates. Foot Ankle Int 2009;30:1161–7.
20. Miller DL, Goswami T. A review of locking compression plate biomechanics and their advantages as internal fixators in fracture healing. Clin Biomech (Bristol, Avon) 2007;22:1049–62.
21. Hazarika S, Chakravarthy J, Cooper J. Minimally invasive locking plate osteosynthesis for fractures of the distal tibia–results in 20 patients. Injury 2006;37: 877–87.
22. Greiwe RM, Archdeacon MT. Locking plate technology: current concepts. J Knee Surg 2007;20:50–5.
23. Perren SM, Russenberger M, Steinemann S, et al. A dynamic compression plate. Acta Orthop Scand Suppl 1969;125:31–41.
24. Gautier E. Mechanics of plate fixation. J Arthroplasty 1994;9:665–6.
25. Miclau T, Remiger A, Tepic S, et al. A mechanical comparison of the dynamic compression plate, limited contact-dynamic compression plate, and point contact fixator. J Orthop Trauma 1995;9:17–22.
26. Farouk O, Krettek C, Miclau T, et al. Minimally invasive plate osteosynthesis: does percutaneous plating disrupt femoral blood supply less than the traditional technique? J Orthop Trauma 1999;13:401–6.
27. Frigg R. Development of the locking compression plate. Injury 2003;34(Suppl 2): B6–10.
28. Kaab MJ, Frenk A, Schmeling A, et al. Locked internal fixator: sensitivity of screw/plate stability to the correct insertion angle of the screw. J Orthop Trauma 2004; 18:483–7.
29. Shereff MJ. Complex fractures of the metatarsals. Orthopedics 1990;13:875–82.
30. Donahue MP, Manoli A 2nd. Technical tip: transverse percutaneous pinning of metatarsal neck fractures. Foot Ankle Int 2004;25:438–9.
31. O'Malley MJ, Hamilton WG, Munyak J. Fractures of the distal shaft of the fifth metatarsal. "Dancer's fracture". Am J Sports Med 1996;24:240–3.
32. Rammelt S, Heineck J, Zwipp H. Metatarsal fractures. Injury 2004;35(Suppl 2): SB77–86.
33. Theodorou DJ, Theodorou SJ, Kakitsubata Y, et al. Fractures of proximal portion of fifth metatarsal bone: anatomic and imaging evidence of a pathogenesis of avulsion of the plantar aponeurosis and the short peroneal muscle tendon. Radiology 2003;226:857–65.
34. Quill GE Jr. Fractures of the proximal fifth metatarsal. Orthop Clin North Am 1995; 26:353–61.

35. Chuckpaiwong B, Queen RM, Easley ME, et al. Distinguishing Jones and prox-imal diaphyseal fractures of the fifth metatarsal. Clin Orthop Relat Res 2008; 466:1966–70.
36. Mindrebo N, Shelbourne KD, Van Meter CD, et al. Outpatient percutaneous screw fixation of the acute Jones fracture. Am J Sports Med 1993;21:720–3.
37. Donley BG, McCollum MJ, Murphy GA, et al. Risk of sural nerve injury with intra-medullary screw fixation of fifth metatarsal fractures: a cadaver study. Foot Ankle Int 1999;20:182–4.
38. Larson CM, Almekinders LC, Taft TN, et al. Intramedullary screw fixation of Jones fractures. Analysis of failure. Am J Sports Med 2002;30:55–60.
39. Ly TV, Coetzee JC. Treatment of primarily ligamentous Lisfranc joint injuries: primary arthrodesis compared with open reduction and internal fixation. A prospective, randomized study. J Bone Joint Surg Am 2006;88:514–20.
40. Henning JA, Jones CB, Sietsema DL, et al. Open reduction internal fixation versus primary arthrodesis for Lisfranc injuries: a prospective randomized study. Foot Ankle Int 2009;30:913–22.
41. Perugia D, Basile A, Battaglia A, et al. Fracture dislocations of Lisfranc's joint treated with closed reduction and percutaneous fixation. Int Orthop 2003;27:30–5.
42. Stavlas P, Roberts CS, Xypnitos FN, et al. The role of reduction and internal fixa-tion of Lisfranc fracture-dislocations: a systematic review of the literature. Int Or-thop 2010;34:1083–91.
43. Harvey EJ, Grujic L, Early JS, et al. Morbidity associated with ORIF of intra-articular calcaneus fractures using a lateral approach. Foot Ankle Int 2001;22: 868–73.
44. Hackstock H, Kolbow H. The percutaneous drill-wire osteosynthesis in intra-articular fractures of the calcaneus. Treatment results. Arch Orthop Unfallchir 1971;71:171–80 [in German].
45. Tornetta P 3rd. The Essex-Lopresti reduction for calcaneal fractures revisited. J Orthop Trauma 1998;12:469–73.
46. Sanders R, Fortin P, DiPasquale T, et al. Operative treatment in 120 displaced in-traarticular calcaneal fractures. Results using a prognostic computed tomog-raphy scan classification. Clin Orthop Relat Res 1993;(290):87–95.
47. Rammelt S, Amlang M, Barthel S, et al. Percutaneous treatment of less severe in-traarticular calcaneal fractures. Clin Orthop Relat Res 2010;468:983–90.
48. Schuberth JM, Cobb MD, Talarico RH. Minimally invasive arthroscopic-assisted reduction with percutaneous fixation in the management of intra-articular calca-neal fractures: a review of 24 cases. J Foot Ankle Surg 2009;48:315–22.
49. Benirschke SK, Kramer PA. Wound healing complications in closed and open calcaneal fractures. J Orthop Trauma 2004;18:1–6.
50. Folk JW, Starr AJ, Early JS. Early wound complications of operative treatment of calcaneus fractures: analysis of 190 fractures. J Orthop Trauma 1999;13: 369–72.
51. Abidi NA, Dhawan S, Gruen GS, et al. Wound-healing risk factors after open reduc-tion and internal fixation of calcaneal fractures. Foot Ankle Int 1998;19:856–61.
52. Schepers T, Van der Stoep A, Van der Avert H, et al. Plantar pressure analysis after percutaneous repair of displaced intra-articular calcaneal fractures. Foot Ankle Int 2008;29:128–35.
53. Comfort TH, Behrens F, Gaither DW, et al. Long-term results of displaced talar neck fractures. Clin Orthop Relat Res 1985;(199):81 7.
54. Vallier HA, Nork SE, Barei DP, et al. Talar neck fractures: results and outcomes. J Bone Joint Surg Am 2004;86:1616–24.

55. Hawkins LG. Fractures of the neck of the talus. J Bone Joint Surg Am 1970;52: 991–1002.
56. Cronier P, Talha A, Massin P. Central talar fractures–therapeutic considerations. Injury 2004;35(Suppl 2):SB10–22.
57. Vallier HA, Nork SE, Benirschke SK, et al. Surgical treatment of talar body fractures. J Bone Joint Surg Am 2004;86(Suppl 1):180–92.
58. Fayazi AH, Reid JS, Juliano PJ. Percutaneous pinning of talar neck fractures. Am J Orthop (Belle Mead NJ) 2002;31:76–8.
59. Pajenda G, Vecsei V, Reddy B, et al. Treatment of talar neck fractures: clinical results of 50 patients. J Foot Ankle Surg 2000;39:365–75.
60. Lee HJ, Kang KS, Kang SY, et al. Percutaneous reduction technique using a Kirschner wire for displaced posterior malleolar fractures. Foot Ankle Int 2009;30:157–9.
61. Ray TD, Nimityongskul P, Anderson LD. Percutaneous intramedullary fixation of lateral malleolus fractures: technique and report of early results. J Trauma 1994;36:669–75.
62. Tornetta P 3rd, Creevy W. Lag screw only fixation of the lateral malleolus. J Orthop Trauma 2001;15:119–21.
63. Raasch WG, Larkin JJ, Draganich LF. Assessment of the posterior malleolus as a restraint to posterior subluxation of the ankle. J Bone Joint Surg Am 1992;74: 1201–6.
64. Bone L, Stegemann P, McNamara K, et al. External fixation of severely comminuted and open tibial pilon fractures. Clin Orthop Relat Res 1993;(292):101–7.
65. Syed MA, Panchbhavi VK. Fixation of tibial pilon fractures with percutaneous cannulated screws. Injury 2004;35:284–9.
66. Collinge C, Protzman R. Outcomes of minimally invasive plate osteosynthesis for metaphyseal distal tibia fractures. J Orthop Trauma 2010;24:24–9.
67. Collinge C, Sanders R, DiPasquale T. Treatment of complex tibial periarticular fractures using percutaneous techniques. Clin Orthop Relat Res 2000;(375): 69–77.
68. Bloomstein L, Schenk R, Grob P. Percutaneous plating of periarticular tibial fractures: a reliable, reproducible technique for controlling plate passage and positioning. J Orthop Trauma 2008;22:566–71.
69. Moller M, Movin T, Granhed H, et al. Acute rupture of tendon Achilles. A prospective randomised study of comparison between surgical and non-surgical treatment. J Bone Joint Surg Br 2001;83:843–8.
70. Lim J, Dalal R, Waseem M. Percutaneous vs. open repair of the ruptured Achilles tendon–a prospective randomized controlled study. Foot Ankle Int 2001;22: 559–68.
71. Tenenbaum S, Dreiangel N, Segal A, et al. The percutaneous surgical approach for repairing acute Achilles tendon rupture: a comprehensive outcome assessment. J Am Podiatr Med Assoc 2010;100:270–5.
72. Ma GW, Griffith TG. Percutaneous repair of acute closed ruptured Achilles tendon: a new technique. Clin Orthop Relat Res 1977;(128):247–55.
73. Gorschewsky O, Vogel U, Schweizer A, et al. Percutaneous tenodesis of the Achilles tendon. A new surgical method for the treatment of acute Achilles tendon rupture through percutaneous tenodesis. Injury 1999;30:315–21.
74. Gorschewsky O, Pitzl M, Putz A, et al. Percutaneous repair of acute Achilles tendon rupture. Foot Ankle Int 2004;25:219–24.

Total Ankle Replacements: An Overview

Lawrence A. DiDomenico, DPM[a,b,c,*], Michelle C. Anania, DPM[c]

KEYWORDS

• Total ankle replacement • Ankle arthroplasty • Ankle arthritis
• Ankle arthrodesis

First performed in the early 1970s, the total ankle replacement (TAR) gives patients who are affected by end-stage ankle arthritis an alternative to fusion. Like an ankle arthrodesis, the purpose of an ankle arthroplasty is to eliminate pain; however, the arthroplasty also looks to maintain function.[1–5] Total joint replacement, whether it is the hip, the knee, or the ankle, involves the removal of the arthritic joint and substituting it with an artificial joint to retain motion. Because of the biomechanics involved at the ankle joint, the TAR is a much more challenging procedure when compared with the hip and knee replacements. In addition, various conditions, if present, add to the level of surgical difficulty and decrease the chance of a successful outcome. These conditions include deformity from posttraumatic arthritis, diabetic neuropathy, and inadequate soft tissue envelope.[4,6,7] Coetzee and DeOrio[8] thought that the TAR will never become as commonplace as the knee and hip replacements because of the level of difficulty and the number of conditions that can adversely affect the outcome.

Since the first TAR was implanted, its short- and long-term benefits have been compared with those of an ankle arthrodesis, the traditional gold standard for end-stage ankle arthritis. Saltzman and colleagues[6] pointed out that the primary indication for both the TAR and the ankle arthrodesis is pain. In their study, they compared the clinical findings of both procedures. They found a better outcome in pain relief and retained motion in those patients who had a TAR at the 2- to 6-year postoperative mark. In another study, the same authors showed a better level of function and a greater level of pain relief in those patients with a TAR compared with those with an arthodesis.[9] Furthermore, Barg and colleagues[10] claimed that most patients with a TAR report favorable outcomes regarding pain relief and ankle function.

[a] Ohio College of Podiatric Medicine, Cleveland, OH, USA
[b] Section of Podiatric Medicine and Surgery, St Elizabeth's Medical Center, Youngstown, OH, USA
[c] Ankle and Foot Care Centers, Youngstown, OH, USA
* Corresponding author. 8175 Market Street, Youngstown, OH 44512.
E-mail address: LD5353@aol.com

Clin Podiatr Med Surg 28 (2011) 727–744
doi:10.1016/j.cpm.2011.08.002
0891-8422/11/$ – see front matter © 2011 Elsevier Inc. All rights reserved.

podiatric.theclinics.com

The short-term results of an ankle fusion are generally very good, but the long-term results are not as clear and tend to be riddled with complications such as pseudoarthrosis, malunion/nonunion, gait abnormalities, and a long period of recovery. The most common complication is the development of arthritis in the adjacent joints, that is, the calcaneocuboid joint, talonavicular joint, subtalar joint, and knee. The subsequent arthritis may necessitate the need for further surgical intervention.[1,9,11–13] Hintermann and colleagues[13] pointed out that the chances of a young patient with an ankle arthrodesis developing premature degenerative arthritis in the hindfoot are very likely. This is because of the increase in the amount of stress and demand on the surrounding joints.[4,13] Lagaay and Schuberth[14] explained the manner the more distal joints compensate changes when the motion is taken away at the ankle, as in the case of a fusion. This has a significant effect on gait.

Because the outcomes of TAR are significantly improving, surgeons who are trained in TAR are more likely to perform a TAR than a fusion. For some surgeons, TAR is actually viewed to be superior over an arthrodesis because of the preserved motion and, more importantly, the decrease in stress and demand on the distal joints.[3,15] The current ankle implants are proving to be a valuable treatment option for those patients with severe arthritis and those who meet the criteria for ankle replacement. Some surgeons now consider an ankle arthrodesis a salvage procedure.[3,11] Even regarding patients with rheumatoid arthritis, Bonnin and colleagues[16] recommended using a TAR over a fusion because of the increased chance of returning to normal or near-normal activity level. Steck and Anderson[17] also recommended a TAR on patients who have already undergone a triple arthrodesis; however, they explained that a TAR can only be performed in those patients in whom a malaligned triple is not the reason for the ankle arthritis. If deformity is present, then the patient will need a pantalar fusion.

ADVANTAGES AND DISADVANTAGES

A major advantage of the TAR is the preservation of ankle motion. However, TAR typically only preserves the current level of motion in the ankle at the time of surgery. Other advantages include the decreased stress across the distal joints, which decreases the risk of developing premature degenerative arthritis; restoration of the dynamics of the ankle; increased comfort and functional recuperation; and having the option to revise the prosthesis or convert the prosthesis to a fusion if the original replacement fails.[4,7,16,18] Bonnin and colleagues[16] discovered that the use of a TAR can actually improve the patient's quality of life. TARs allow the return to recreational and/or light-impact activities and sports. A return to high-impact activities and sports, however, is not recommended and highly unlikely.

The risk of TAR includes significant complications and failure that may still then necessitate an arthrodesis.[16] Patients who experience significant complications such as deep infection and wound problems require significant intervention, and the subsequent need for a below-knee amputation is a possibility.

INDICATIONS AND CONTRAINDICATIONS

TAR is indicated for patients with end-stage ankle arthritis. The pathologic condition of the arthritis can be either primary or secondary. Secondary osteoarthritis, that is, posttraumatic arthritis, accounts for most of the cases of ankle arthritis. Posttraumatic arthritis is the leading cause of ankle arthritis and can be because of a history of a fracture involving the ankle joint or even a history of ankle sprains leading to chronic lateral ankle instability. Chronic inflammation in the ankle joint because of gout, rheumatoid arthritis, psoriatic arthritis, infection, hemophilia, hemochromatosis, and osteochondritis dissecans can also lead to severe damage of the ankle joint.[3,4,8,17,19-26] Patients with hemophilia typically have a target joint in which recurrent episodes of hemarthrosis eventually cause severe damage to the joint. Typically, the standard of care for a patient with hemophiliac arthritis is an ankle fusion; however, the TAR is proving to be a valuable option although it is still considered controversial.[11] Charcot neuroarthropathy and tumors can also lead to arthritis; however, at present, these conditions are contraindicated for TAR surgery.

Increasing comfort with the implant designs and techniques is making TAR a more viable treatment option in patients with pain because of a failed ankle arthrodesis. Whether failure is because of a nonunion, malunion, continued pain after fusion, or pain associated with osteoarthritis of the adjacent joints, TAR may be an option.[27] However, in this patient population, it is mandatory for the patient to have their fibula intact when the arthrodesis was performed. Revisions in the case without the fibula can have a significant negative effect on outcomes and, therefore, are not recommended.

One of the most critical steps in achieving a successful outcome is proper patient selection. There are no clear-cut guidelines regarding the inclusion and exclusion criteria.[8,17] General indications include an older patient, one who is near the age of 55 years, with a low physical demand, good bone stock, intact neurovascular status, an intact immune system, good alignment of the ankle, and no ligamentous laxity.[17]

Van Den Heuvel and colleagues[3] divided the contraindications for a TAR into absolute and relative.

Absolute contraindications
 1. An active or recent infection in or around the ankle joint.
 2. A neuropathic joint, which may lead to further breakdown and instability.
 3. Poor bone stock of the talus because of severe osteoporosis or avascular necrosis of more than 50% of the talar body.
 4. Poor quality of the skin and soft tissue envelope surrounding the ankle, including skin disease, which will lead to a greater chance of wound dehiscence and infection.
 5. Any type of neurologic dysfunction of the affected limb such as paralysis.
 6. Severe irreducible malalignment of the leg, ankle, or foot.
 7. Chronic ankle instability.
 8. Peripheral vascular disease. Many surgeons do not recommend surgery on patients with digital pressures less than 70 mm Hg.
 9. Noncompliance.
10. Chronic pain syndrome.[1,3,4,8,23-25]

Suggestions as to the cutoff point for performing a TAR in the presence of a varus or valgus hindfoot deformity range from 10° to 30° in either direction.[1] Many surgeons consider a varus or valgus hindfoot deformity of more than 20° to be an absolute contraindication for a TAR.[1,3,4,8,20,21,23,28] Some surgeons suggest stricter guidelines, that is, the degree of deformity should not be greater than 10° to 15° of either varus or valgus.[29] Coetzee recalled a series of 200 patients who had a TAR with a preoperative varus deformity of more than 20°. Postoperatively, the failure rate was 50% and the failed TARs were converted to an arthrodesis. Because of the unacceptably high failure rate, the author avoids performing a TAR on any patient with more than 20°

of varus deformity.[21] Mendicino and colleagues[4] first observed the ankle joint as being either congruent or incongruent. If the patient has more than 15° of varus or valgus deformity in a congruent ankle joint, or if there is more than 10° of varus or valgus deformity in an incongruent joint, then a TAR should be avoided. They explained further that any deformity that will not allow the foot to be plantigrade will cause the implant to fail because of the increase in stress and strain across the device; thus, a TAR should also be avoided in these cases. If malalignment is present, it needs to be corrected either before a TAR, making this a 2-stage procedure, or at the time of the TAR, a 1-stage procedure.[3]

Regarding relative contraindications, Steck and Anderson[17] strongly advised considering an alternate form of treatment if multiple relative contraindications exist with a patient.

Examples of relative contraindications:
1. Young age
2. High physical demands
3. Obesity
4. Diabetes
5. Previous open ankle fracture or dislocation
6. History of osteomyelitis that was successfully treated
7. Malnutrition
8. Smoker
9. Immunosuppression therapy, that is, long-term steroid use.

In their study of patients with a mean age of 44 years or younger who had a TAR, Spirt and colleagues[30] found these younger patients to be 1.45 times likely to require further surgery. In addition, the risk of failure was more than 2.5 times greater in the younger patients compared with the patients older than 54 years. Lagaay and Schuberth[14] discovered in their study a significant association between high patient satisfaction levels and those patients aged at least 60 years with a body mass index of less than 30. However, they explained that the level of satisfaction may be related more to the length of time a patient has been in pain than to the actual age of the patient. For example, a 65-year-old patient who has been in pain for 20 years may report a higher level of satisfaction than a 40-year-old patient who has been in pain for 5 years. Kofoed[25] did not consider young age to be a contraindication; however, the patient must be made aware of the implant's inability to tolerate high-impact forces associated with running and jumping. The age of the patient is associated with the level of physical demand. Younger patients usually have higher physical demands. The older patient tends to have a lower physical demand, which means less force and impact across the implant and the less chance of failure.

Absolute contraindications also exist when converting an ankle fusion into an ankle arthroplasty, which include the presence of clubfoot, Charcot neuroarthropathy, poor circulation, and large scars on the medial aspect of the ankle along with severe compromise of the soft tissue structures. Relative contraindications include an absent distal fibula, valgus deformity, severe dorsal soft tissue contractures secondary to prolonged immobilization, and leg shortening greater than 3 cm (**Fig. 1**A, B).[13]

BIOMECHANICS

Because of the biomechanics involved at the level of the ankle, one cannot compare an ankle replacement with a replacement of the hip or knee. The ankle needs to be able to withstand 500% of the patient's body weight during the normal gait cycle on

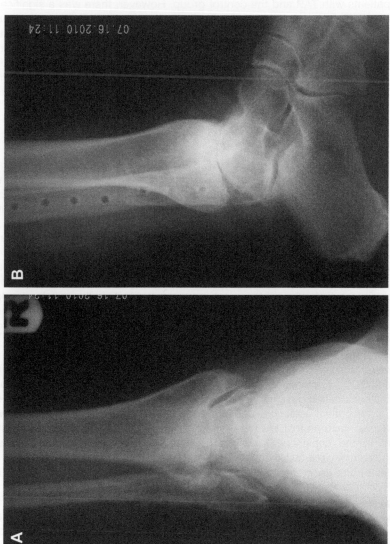

Fig. 1. (*A*) and (*B*) Demonstrating a patient who is an ideal candidate for TAR. The patient is affected by posttraumatic arthritis and is elderly and thin, and his activities consist of light physical demand with no significant deformity.

a much smaller surface area. The slightest variation in the surface alignment of the ankle joint can lead to implant failure. Joint incongruity can cause polyethylene wear and osteolysis.[31] Lee and colleagues[32] performed a study to examine the patient's static and dynamic postural imbalance 1 year after TAR. In the motor impairment arm of the study, patients with TAR demonstrated a decrease in motor control. In the sensory impairment arm of the study, there was no difference in proprioception between patients with TAR and the control group. However, there was a significant degree of dynamic postural imbalance with the patients with TAR. These patients were found to rely more on hip function to keep their balance. The authors surmised that this may be related to the decrease in muscle strength at the leg and ankle along with the decrease in reflexes at the ankle. Morgan and colleagues[33] described the results of a gait analysis study conducted by Piviou and colleagues on patients with TAR, which showed a better overall gait analysis regarding pattern, timing, and distribution of ground reaction force compared with patients with an ankle arthrodesis.

DESIGNS

Lord and Marotte introduced the first TAR in the early 1970s.[3,34] The implant had a ball-and-socket–type design based on the hip replacement. Of the 25 patients who underwent the TAR procedure, 18 patients failed. Because of this unacceptably high failure rate, they recommended fusing the ankle joint than trying to replace it.[3] Later, first-generation implants were constrained or unconstrained, cemented, 2-component systems consisting of a polyethylene concave tibial component and a metal convex talar component.[2,3,24] These implants acted like a hinge joint, allowing motion in only 1 plane. The constrained version generated force on the cement-bone interface, which led to loosening of the implant,[1,4,17,18] whereas the early unconstrained designs, which allowed the most movement, relied on the collateral ankle ligaments for support. This unconstrained version was prone to displacement because of the inherent instability.[1,35] Other common complications of the first-generation implants were subsidence and osteolysis.[17,35]

The survival rate at less than 5 years for the first-generation implants was 80% to 85%; however, long-term outcomes proved to be very poor. The revision rate was upward of 40%.[3,17] Factors contributing to the high failure rate include the nonanatomic or malconstrained designs, the use of cement, the need for aggressive bone resection, poor patient selection, and poor surgical technique.[4,9] Van Den Heuvel and colleagues[3] thought that the high rate of failure could be attributed to the use of cement in the constrained designs. Because of the poor outcomes, first-generation designs were quickly abandoned and are no longer in use.[12,36]

Examples of first-generation designs are the Conaxial ankle replacement and the Mayo TAR.[3,5]

The high failure rate of the first-generation implants led to the development of the second-generation implants.[37] Technical improvements included a less-constrained design to decrease the amount of shear and torsion, the need for less bone resection, and uncemented designs. The tibial and talar components were given stems and pegs to assist with stability and load distribution by allowing bony ingrowth than relying on cement.[3,4,7] With new implant designs, a new set of complications arose, including failure of the polyethylene insert, instability, impingement, and component dislocation.[4]

The second-generation implants are uncemented, 2-component, polyethylene-on-metal designs that can be divided into 1 of 2 types. The first type is a 2-component, fixed-bearing implant in which the polyethylene insert is fixed to the tibial component.

This gives the implant 1 point of articulation between the talar and the tibial components. This type of fixed or semiconstrained design is used in the United States at present. The second type of second-generation implant is the 3-component, mobile-bearing implant. This type has a polyethylene insert that is not fixed to either the tibial or the talar component. It is free to move between the 2 components, thus giving the implant 2 points of articulation. This freely moving meniscus greatly reduces the amount of shearing on any 1 surface. Also, the lack of constraints on the insert reduces the amount of wear on the insert.[1–3,17,35] The Scandanavian total ankle replacement (STAR) is at present the only Food and Drug Administration–approved mobile-bearing implant used in the United States.

The STAR implant was designed by Dr Hakon Kofoed in 1978 and first came into use in the early 1980s. The original design was a 2-component, cemented, unconstrained, fixed-bearing implant. Because of the high rate of loosening associated with this design, many modifications took place. The STAR ankle implant is now a 3-component, uncemented, mobile-bearing device that requires minimal bone resection. The newer design decreases the rotational stress at the bone-implant interface and is the most commonly used ankle replacement system in Europe.[3,4,35,37]

The Buechel-Pappas ankle implant was introduced in the United States in 1981. At present it is an uncemented, 3-component, mobile-bearing device. The talar component has a fin-type fixation design that reduces the amount of subsidence.[3,37] This implant is not available in the United States at present.

The Agility ankle implant was introduced in 1984 by Frank Alvine, MD. This was the first and most popular implant of its generation in early 2000s in the United States and is a fixed-bearing, semiconstrained design. This ankle implant, unlike any other, requires a fusion of the syndesmosis to allow load sharing through the fibula. The fusion improves overall stability and provides support to the tibial component. This implant also requires the use of an external fixator for distraction during surgery.[3,8,36–38]

The idea of soft tissue balancing led to the development of the third-generation designs. These implants place more emphasis on stability by relying on the collateral ligaments. Most of these designs are noncemented, 3-component, mobile-bearing implants that require minimal bone resection. The polyethylene insert is not fixed to either component.[2,3,33,34,36]

Initially, these implants had a flat tibial component and a convex talar component. This design created a lot of instability in the ankle, which ultimately led to implant failure. The latest versions copy the natural movements of the ankle joint, thus decreasing the amount of strain on the ligaments. These designs have a talar component that mimics the natural anatomic shape of the talus and a tibial component that is convex and spherical than flat. This is found to be compatible with the ankle ligaments.[11,23,34]

The metal tibial and talar components are made of either cobalt-chromium or a combination of cobalt-chromium and titanium. Hydroxyapatite is used as a coating to facilitate bone fixation in the implants used in Europe. The implants used in the United States and Canada have a titanium porous coating.[3,39] Compared with the second-generation implants, the third-generation implants have a second interface between the tibial component and the polyethylene insert, which allows for better adaptation to changes in position, thus decreasing the degree of abnormal loading on the ligaments and the degree of wear on the insert.[11]

There are approximately 23 different types of third-generation implants in use worldwide at present. One example is the BOX ankle, described by Giannini and colleagues.[23] This implant has tibial and talar component shapes that are nonanatomic, and the polyethylene insert is fully conforming. This version can only be used in patients with stable ankle ligaments because the implant allows the ligaments to remain isometric during passive motion (**Figs. 2–4**).[23,37]

PREOPERATIVE DEFORMITIES

When ankle deformities, most importantly a varus or valgus deformity, are present preoperatively, they must be corrected before or in conjunction with the insertion of a TAR to ensure a successful outcome. Because of the location of the foot to the ankle and the role the foot plays in balance and alignment, a stable plantigrade foot will have a positive effect on the success rate of the TAR.[8,21]

The ipsilateral lower limb of the affected ankle needs to be thoroughly examined. Any bony deformity above, at, or below the level of the ankle joint can adversely affect the alignment of the ankle and the function of the TAR.[1,17,21] Failure to correct any preoperative deformity leads to premature failure of the implant because of edge loading, bearing subluxation, and polyethylene wear.[22]

Many surgeons agree that the presence of either a varus or a valgus deformity makes the TAR procedure much more challenging and the outcome less success-ful.[8,21] If a preoperative varus or valgus deformity is not corrected, this increases the risk of implant failure because of instability, implant tilting, bearing subluxation, or bearing dislocation.[29] There is a wide disparity, and many varying opinions are in the literature of the correctable upper limits of frontal-plane deformities. Patients with a varus or valgus deformity of more than 10° are at a greater risk of developing instability and bearing subluxation. In addition, a study by Haskell and Mann revealed a 10 times greater risk of developing edge loading in an incongruent joint.[1] Hobson and colleagues[15] demonstrated that when the proper steps are taken to surgically correct the varus or valgus deformity at the time of the TAR, patients with a preoperative deformity of up to 30° are not at an increased risk of developing postoperative complications and implant failure. The authors conceded that still the most common type of failure especially in patients with more than 20° of deformity is instability. For any deformity greater than 30°, a fusion is recommended. Coetzee[21] recommended an arthrodesis in those ankles with greater than 20° of deformity. Fifty percent of the patients who had a TAR performed in an ankle with more than 20° of preoperative varus deformity went on to failure within 3 years. Wood and colleagues[28] recommended a fusion when the varus or valgus deformity is more than 20°. Anders and

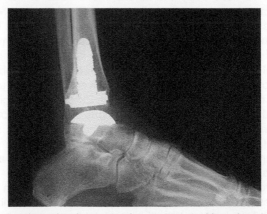

Fig. 2. A postoperative lateral radiograph of an in-bone ankle arthroplasty.

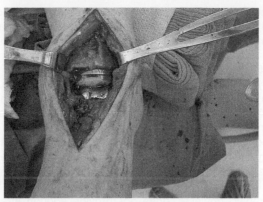

Fig. 3. An intraoperative view demonstrating an operative view of a Salto Tolaris ankle implant after insertion into the distal tibial-talar joint.

colleagues[19] also advised doing an ankle fusion over a TAR in patients with a severe varus or valgus deformity.

Recently, Shock and colleagues[40] demonstrated a stepwise approach for consistent correction for coronal-plane deformities.

Regarding valgus deformities, Coetzee and DeOrio[8] stated that mild to moderate cases can usually be corrected with a medial calcaneal osteotomy and a repair of

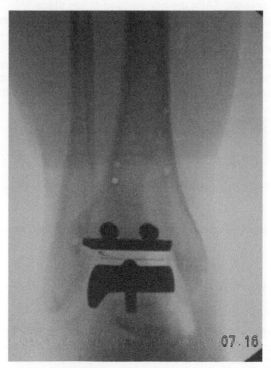

Fig. 4. An intraoperative anteroposterior view after insertion of a STAR implant.

the medial soft tissue structures including the deltoid ligament. In more severe cases, a double-stranded allograft is needed to reconstruct the deltoid ligament. In patients with rheumatoid arthritis, a valgus ankle is reported as the most common deformity, found in as much as 29% of patients who have had rheumatoid arthritis for more than 5 years (**Fig. 5**).[1,25]

A varus deformity can be caused by lateral instability, bony erosion, or a combination of both. Correction of a varus deformity should take place in a proximal-to-distal direction, making the TAR the last procedure performed.[21] A stepwise approach has been developed by Alvine to classify the degree of varus deformity and how it should be surgically managed. Stage 1 is a mild deformity because of medial bone erosion. The varus deformity can be eliminated with the tibial bone cuts. Once the tibial component is in place, the surgeon should test for medial and lateral instability and make any needed repairs. The instability can usually be corrected with a lateral ligament repair. A simple Broström repair, however, does not provide enough strength to maintain stability. Stage 2 deformities have a combination of bony erosion of the medial malleolus and contracture of the medial soft tissue structures. Large osteophytes are also noted in the lateral gutter of the ankle joint. Multiple corrective procedures need to be performed before the TAR to eliminate the varus deformity, restore motion by removing the osteophytes, and restore stability. If the medial soft tissue structures are tight, a release of the deep deltoid ligament or a distal sliding osteotomy of the medial malleolus is performed. If a varus deformity is still present in the hindfoot even after the ankle joint has been mobilized and realigned, then a lateral closing wedge calcaneal osteotomy needs to be performed. Stage 3 deformities are characterized by severe instability along with secondary deformities. These patients require not only an ankle arthrodesis but also a fusion of the subtalar joint because of the degree of arthritis present. TARs are not advised at this stage.[8,21]

Kim and colleagues[29] developed algorithms for moderate to severe ankle varus deformities to assist in proper surgical correction. The first step is to identify the varus deformity as either congruent or incongruent, which is determined by the degree of talar tilt. A talar tilt of less than 10° is considered congruent, whereas that of more than 10° is incongruent. In congruent deformities, the ankle mortise is usually tilted along with the talus. To correct this, the tibia is cut to neutralize the mortise along

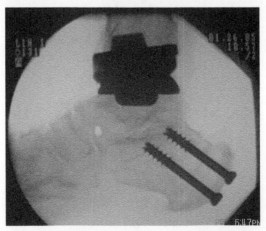

Fig. 5. An interoperative lateral radiograph demonstrating an Agility ankle implant. The patient had a preoperative calcaneal varus deformity; thus, a lateral slide calcaneal osteotomy was performed.

with a medial soft tissue release. Incongruent deformities are because of contracture of the medial soft tissue structures. In these cases, the ankle mortise is properly aligned. Balancing the lateral soft tissue structures results in a neutral ankle.

When converting an ankle arthrodesis into an ankle arthroplasty, Hintermann and colleagues[27] recommended examining the surrounding joints for arthritic changes. If arthritis is present, fusion of the adjacent joints should take place before the takedown of the ankle fusion. Other preoperative abnormalities, if present, that need to be surgically addressed before a TAR include medial and lateral ligament insufficiency, an equinus deformity, and malalignment of the calcaneus.

COMPLICATIONS

According to Steck and Anderson,[17] complications from a TAR procedure occur because of 1 of 3 reasons: poor patient selection, inexperience on behalf of the surgeon, or surgical error. The TAR has a steep learning curve, and the success of the implant depends on the level of the surgeon's experience. Also one must keep in mind that every new implant has its own learning curve. Lee and colleagues[41] explained that the rate of complication decreases as the surgeon's experience with the implant increases. The authors described a study of 50 patients who underwent TAR using the Hintegra device (Life Sciences Plainsboro, NJ, USA). The first 25 patients had a higher incidence of complications compared with the last 25 patients. The chance of a successful outcome also increases as the surgeon's experience increases.[10,17,19,41,42]

Performing a TAR on the proper patient also aids in decreasing the risk of postoperative complications and in increasing the chance of a successful outcome. Therefore, patients should meet strict criteria through strict inclusion guidelines and a thorough perioperative workup. Proper surgical technique and choosing the proper implant also play an important role in achieving a successful outcome and in decreasing the rate of complications.[3,4] Certain conditions, however, are prone to a higher complication rate because of the pathologic condition of the arthritis. Bai and colleagues[43] found the rate of complication to be higher in patients with posttraumatic arthritis compared with those with primary osteoarthritis.

Glazebrook and colleagues[12] thought that the rate of a complication is not an accurate measure of its severity; therefore, they divided the complications of a TAR into 3 groups based on its effect on the outcome, that is, its rate of failure. The 3 groups are low-, medium-, and high-grade complications. Low-grade complications have minimal risk of causing TAR failure, and examples include intraoperative fractures and superficial wound issues. Medium-grade complications cause failure of the implant less than 50% of the time and include technical error, subsidence, and postoperative fractures. High-grade complications cause failure of the implant more than 50% of the time and include deep infection and aseptic loosening.

Wound complications can be categorized as either major or minor. Minor wounds tend to be superficial, require local care only, and pose no threat to the implant. Necrosis of the skin edges is considered a minor wound complication. A major wound is an infection of the deep soft tissue layers that poses a threat to the implant. To decrease the incidence of wound complications, the surgeon should limit the amount of dissection, take care when using retraction, and limit the degree of plantar flexion at the ankle postoperatively, that is, keep the ankle in a neutral position.[17,27] Deep infections need to be handled promptly. The necrotic tissue needs debridement, and cultures need to be taken for proper intravenous antibiotic coverage. Deep infections can lead to septic loosening of the implant, which results in its removal and the insertion of an antibiotic cement spacer. Any type of revision is held off until the infection is completely eradicated. Infection rates range from 0.5% to 3.5% and are higher among an ankle arthroplasty than a knee or hip arthroplasty.[11,19,36]

Subluxation of the polyethylene insert, also known as edge loading, decreases the amount of contact between the insert and the metal components. This causes polyethylene wear particles to buildup, leading to osteolysis. The wear particles stimulate a macrophage-mediated cystic response in the bone. The inflammation mediators, specifically interleukin 1 and 2, tumor necrosis factor, and prostaglandin, inhibit osteoblasts and stimulate osteoclastic activity. Osteolysis is seen on a radiograph as lucent areas in the talus, tibia, and/or the fibula. Mechanical lysis is also known as ballooning lysis and presents early in the postoperative course. This type of lysis is because of remodeling of the tibia and stress shielding and is not a threat to the implant. Expansile lysis occurs late in the postoperative course and is progressive to the point in which bone grafting is needed to counteract any weakness in the bone. This type of lysis is usually because of an abnormal wear.[17,20,44,45] Besse and colleagues[20] evaluated the rate of osteolysis when using the ankle evolutive system (AES). They observed a higher rate of osteolysis, which led to a higher rate of subsidence. Because of this finding, the authors have discontinued using this system. Koivu and colleagues[44] found the risk of osteolysis to be more than 3 times higher in patients with the AES implant because of the dual-coating, titanium-hydroxyapatite coating than in those with implants that have only the hydroxyapatite coating. Because of the concerns regarding the high rate of osteolysis when using the AES implant, the manufacturer has withdrawn the implant from use.[33]

Subsidence of the prosthetic components requires revision of the implant, which can be because of poor bone quality, overly aggressive bone resection, improper implantation of the device, use of a device that is too small, and sepsis.[1,17]

Loosening of the implant is caused by a failure of bony ingrowth on the implant or an interruption of bony ingrowth, also known as aseptic loosening. Patients complain of pain and have a dark halo around the implant. The halo is because of the lack of bony ingrowth.[17] Loosening of the talar component may be because of malalignment, poor bone quality, noncompliance, and malrotation of the talus. Talar malrotation can lead to an increase in polyethylene wear and an increase in rotational torque.[31]

Fractures of the medial and lateral malleolus can show up either early or late in the postoperative course and are the result of surgical error. Early fractures are often the result of surgeon error by commission. Late fractures are usually the result of a surgeon's negligence, resulting in an improperly balanced ankle.[20] The medial malleolus is commonly fractured. One or 2 Kirschner wires can be driven into the medial malleolus before making the horizontal cuts, which prevents overzealous cuts, thus decreasing the risk of fracture. This same technique can also be used to prevent fractures on the lateral malleolus (**Figs. 6** and **7**).[27,29]

Malalignment can be prevented with careful preoperative planning and the use of fluoroscopy throughout the procedure. When present, malalignment will cause an increase in the amount of force generated between the metal component and the bone, which in turn leads to osteolysis because of the buildup of polyethylene wear particles.[27,29]

Sensory deficits and nerve damage occur if any 1 of the nerves that cross the ankle joint is lacerated during surgery. Traction injuries can also occur because of nerve exposure. The superficial peroneal nerve and its branches are at greatest risk for injury because of its close proximity to the anterior incision. Careful dissection is needed to prevent injury to this nerve and any other nerve that is in or near the area of dissection.[17,27,36]

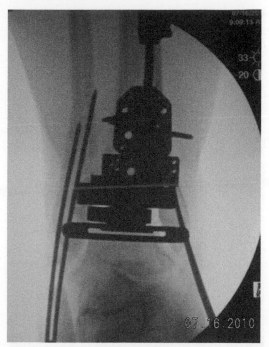

Fig. 6. An intraoperative view demonstrating the use of 2 Kirschner wires on each of the medial and lateral malleolus to avoid fracturing the malleolus before making the tibial bone cuts.

A complication that is unique to the Agility implant is nonunion of the syndesmosis. A nonunion can increase the risk of malalignment of the tibial component, subsidence, and osteolysis. If the nonunion persists for more than 6 months, revision is needed.[7,8]

Kim and colleagues[46] found that patients who had a TAR performed simultaneously with a hindfoot fusion were at a greater risk for instability and dislocation, whereas those who had the TAR and the hindfoot procedures done as a 2-stage process were at a greater risk of developing complications with the soft tissue, such as scarring and bony impingement. In another study, Kim and colleagues[46] noticed an increase in the degree of osteolysis in patients who had a TAR in association with a hindfoot fusion compared with that in those who did not have a hindfoot fusion. This may have an adverse effect on the long-term success of the TAR.

Other complications that can occur with a TAR procedure are deep vein thrombosis, damage to the flexor hallucis longus tendon, and damage to the proprioceptors, which will lead to problems with postural balance (**Fig. 8**A–C).[1,27,32]

CLINICAL OUTCOMES AND SURVIVAL RATES

Barg and colleagues[42] thought that because of the favorable mid- and long-term results, a TAR is recommended in patients with rheumatoid arthritis and posttraumatic arthritis. In patients with hemophilic arthritis, the results are promising enough that they recommend a TAR over an arthrodesis. In a study of patients with hemophilia who had a TAR, all patients experienced a significant decrease in pain. Fifty percent of these patients went on to become completely pain free.

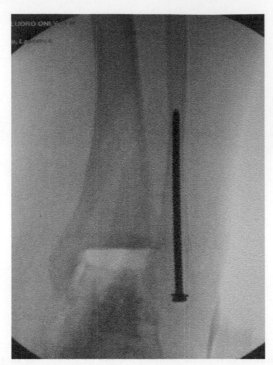

Fig. 7. An interoperative view using a 4-mm cortical screw for repair of a fibula fracture.

Barg and colleagues[10] performed simultaneous bilateral TARs on patients and noted that they had a significant decrease in pain; however, the mean pain score was higher compared with that of the unilateral group.

When analyzing TAR survival rates, Gougoulias and colleagues[24] advised against taking in the data at face value. Much of the information reported may be from the inventors of the implant, which gives a higher survival rate simply because of the familiarity with the implant.

The failure rate for first-generation implants was as high as 36%. For second-generation implants, the midterm results fair better, with a 5-year survival rate of 78% to 93% and a 10-year survival rate of 76% to 80%.[35]

Anders and colleagues[19] showed that consisting of a mid-term analysis of 93 TAR procedures performed with the AES implant, the 5-year survival rate was 90%. Besse and colleagues[20] had a 96% survival rate at 40 months postoperatively using the AES system in 50 ankles. However, because of the high rate of cyst formation and the risk of mechanical failure, the authors refrained from using this device.

Coetzee and DeOrio[8] had a survival rate of 80% in 300 ankles using the Agility implant. They went on to explain that Wood and colleagues had a 5-year survival rate of 93% using the STAR in 200 ankles. Doets and colleagues[47] had a survival rate of 84% at 8 years postoperatively on 93 implants.[1] Patients with rheumatoid arthritis also have good survival rates with TAR procedures. DiDomenico and colleagues[1] pointed out that Fevang and colleagues had a survival rate of 89% in patients with rheumatoid arthritis with a TAR at the 5-year follow-up and 76% at the 10-year follow-up. San Giovanni and colleagues[48] performed 31 TARs on patients with rheumatoid arthritis using the Buechel-Pappas implant. The survival rate was 93% at the 8.3-year average follow-up.[1]

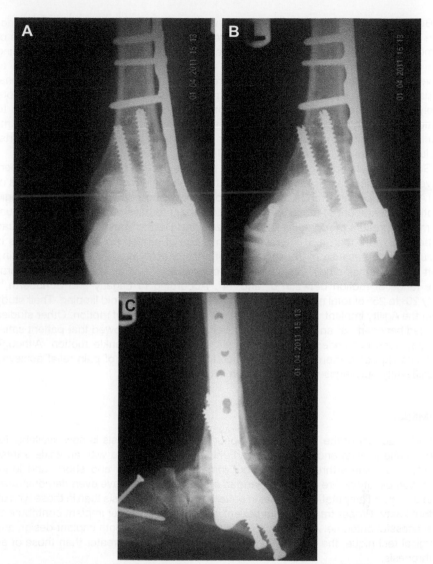

Fig. 8. Anteroposterior (*A*), lateral (*B*), and medial oblique (*C*) radiographic views of an ankle implant converted to an arthrodesis after trauma approximately 6 years after successful implant of an Agility implant. The trauma fractured the talus; therefore, this was converted to a tibal, talar, calcaneal arthrodesis using a femoral locking plate.

EXPECTATIONS

For a successful outcome, the surgeon must use the proper indications, proper patient selection, a well-designed implant, the lifespan of the implant regarding the patient's age, and the proper instruments. The surgeon must also take into account the patient's current level of activity and his or her expected level of function postoperatively.[14,16,19]

Bonnin and colleagues[16] explained that the patient's postoperative level of satisfaction relies heavily on whether his or her preoperative expectations were met. It is of utmost importance that the patient has realistic expectations and goals regarding the overall outcome. The authors further explained that younger patients tend to have unreasonably high expectations regarding their postoperative functional capacity. This is usually because younger patients tend to be more active and more likely to be affected by posttraumatic arthritis. The surgeon must clearly explain to patients that they can expect to participate in light recreational activities and nonimpact sports postoperatively. On the other hand, high-impact activities and sports, including any activity involving running and jumping, are unrealistic.

Gougoulias and colleagues[24] stated that patients need to be made aware preoperatively that an increase in range of motion at the ankle joint is not one of the benefits of a TAR. Postoperative range of motion should never be compared with physiologic motion. The amount of motion a patient can expect to have depends on the amount of motion present preoperatively.[8,14] Coetzee and DeOrio[8] pointed out that one can expect no more than a 5° improvement in range of motion postoperatively. This is thought to be because of the degree of stiffness or laxity present in the surrounding soft tissue. In their study, Gougoulias and colleagues[24] had an improved postoperative range of motion between 0° and 14°. According to Lagaay and Schuberth,[14] only 20° to 25° of total motion is needed at the ankle joint to avoid limping. Their study with the Agility implant was approximately 23° of total range of motion. Other studies ranged between 18° and 36° postoperatively. The authors showed that patient satisfaction does not necessarily correlate with the degree of ankle motion. Although patients expected more motion postoperatively, the amount of pain relief achieved significantly outweighs what little motion is gained.

SUMMARY

With the advent of the TAR, a viable option over an arthrodesis is now available for those patients with end-stage ankle arthritis. When compared with an ankle arthroplasty, the ankle arthrodesis has poor long-term outcomes and short- and long-term complications are common. Haddad and colleagues[49] have even demonstrated that the rate of amputation is higher in patients with anarthrodesis than in those with an arthroplasty. Proper training, strict patient selection, and proper implant contribute to a successful outcome. As advances continue to be made in both implant design and surgical technique, the benefits of a TAR are proving to be greater than those of an arthrodesis.

REFERENCES

1. DiDomenico L, Treadwell J, Cain L. Total ankle arthroplasty in the rheumatoid patient. Clin Podiatr Med Surg 2010;27:295–311.
2. Goldberg A, Sharp R, Cooke P. Ankle replacement: current practice of foot & ankle surgeons in the United Kingdom. Foot Ankle Int 2009;30:950–4.
3. Van Den Heuvel A, Van Bouwel S, Dereymaeker G. Total ankle replacement design evolution and results. Acta Orthop Belg 2010;76:150–61.
4. Mendicino R, Catanzariti A, Shadrick D. The STAR total ankle replacement. Foot Ankle Quarterly 2010;21:157–66.
5. Gougoulias N, Khanna A, Maffulli N. History and evolution in total ankle arthroplasty. Br Med Bull 2009;89:111–51.

6. Saltzman C, Kadoko R, Suh J. Treatment of isolated ankle osteoarthritis with arthrodesis or the total ankle replacement: a comparison of early outcomes. Clin Orthop Surg 2010;2:1–7.

7. Total ankle replacement for degenerative ankle disease. Supplement to OR Manager 2010;26(4).

8. Coetzee J, DeOrio J. Total ankle replacement systems available in the United States. Instr Course Lect 2010;59:367–74.

9. Saltzman C, Mann R, Ahrens J, et al. Prospective controlled trial of STAR total ankle replacement versus ankle fusion: initial results. Foot Ankle Int 2009;30:579–96.

10. Barg A, Knupp M, Hintermann B. Simultaneous bilateral versus unilateral total ankle replacement. A patient-based comparison of pain relief, quality of life and functional outcome. J Bone Joint Surg Br 2010;92:1659–63.

11. Barg A, Elsner A, Chuckpaiwong B, et al. Insert position in three-component total ankle replacement. Foot Ankle Int 2010;31:754–9.

12. Glazebrook M, Arsenault K, Dunbar M. Evidence-based classification of complications in total ankle arthroplasty. Foot Ankle Int 2009;30:945–9.

13. Hintermann B, Barg A, Knupp M, et al. Conversion of painful ankle arthrodesis to total ankle arthroplasty. J Bone Joint Surg Am 2009;91:850–8.

14. Lagaay P, Schuberth J. Analysis of ankle range of motion and functional outcome following total ankle arthroplasty. J Foot Ankle Surg 2010;49:147–51.

15. Hobson S, Karantana A, Dhar S. Total ankle replacement in patients with significant pre-operative deformity of the hindfoot. J Bone Joint Surg Br 2009;91:481–6.

16. Bonnin M, Laurent J, Casillas M. Ankle function and sports activity after total ankle arthroplasty. Foot Ankle Int 2009;30:933–44.

17. Steck J, Anderson J. Total ankle arthroplasty: indications and avoiding complications. Clin Podiatr Med Surg 2009;26:303–24.

18. Van der Heide H, Schutte B, Louwerens J, et al. Total ankle prostheses in rheumatoid arthropathy. Outcome in 52 patients followed for 1-9 years. Acta Orthop 2009;80:440–4.

19. Anders H, Knutson K, Johan L, et al. The AES total ankle replacement. A mid-term analysis of 93 cases. Foot Ankle Surg 2010;16:61–4.

20. Besse J, Brito N, Lienhart C. Clinical evaluation and radiographic assessment of bone lysis of the AES total ankle replacement. Foot Ankle Int 2009;30:964–75.

21. Coetzee J. Surgical strategies: lateral ligament reconstruction as part of the management of varus ankle deformity with ankle replacement. Foot Ankle Int 2010;31:267–74.

22. Frigg A, Nigg B, Hinz L, et al. Clinical relevance of hindfoot alignment view in total ankle replacement. Foot Ankle Int 2010;31:871–9.

23. Giannini S, Romagnoli M, O'Connor J, et al. Total ankle replacement compatible with ligament function produces mobility, good clinical scores, and low complication rates. An early clinical assessment. Clin Orthop Relat Res 2010;468:2746–53.

24. Gougoulias N, Khanna A, Maffulli N. How successful are current ankle replacements? A systematic review of the literature. Clin Orthop Relat Res 2010;468:199–208.

25. Kofoed H. Concept and use of the Scandinavian total ankle replacement. Foot Ankle Spec 2009;2:89–94.

26. Margolis D, Allen-Taylor L, Hoffstad O, et al. Intermediate and long-term outcomes of total ankle arthroplasty and ankle arthrodesis. A systematic review of the literature. Diabet Med 2004;22:172–6.

27 Hintermann B, Barg A, Knupp M, et al. Conversion of painful ankle arthrodesis to total ankle arthroplastyh Surgical technique. J Bone Joint Surg Am 2010; 92(Suppl 1):55–66.

28. Wood P, Karski M, Watmough P. Total ankle replacementh The results of 100 mobility total ankle replacements. J Bone Joint Surg Br 2010;92:958–62.
29. Kim B, Choi W, Kim Y, et al. Total ankle replacement in moderate to severe varus deformity of the ankle. J Bone Joint Surg Br 2009;91:1183–90.
30. Spirt A, Assal M, Hansen S Jr. Complications and failure after total ankle arthroplasty. J Bone Joint Surg Am 2004;86:1172–8.
31. Fukuda T, Haddad S, Ren Y, et al. Impact of talar component rotation on contact pressure after total ankle arthroplasty: a cadaveric study. Foot Ankle Int 2010;31: 404–11.
32. Lee K, Park Y, Song E, et al. Static and dynamic postural balance after successful mobile-bearing total ankle arthroplasty. Arch Phys Med Rehabil 2010;91:519–22.
33. Morgan S, Brooke B, Harris N. Total ankle replacement by the Ankle Evolution System. Medium-term outcome. J Bone Joint Surg Br 2010;92:61–5.
34. Affatato S, Taddei P, Leardini A, et al. Wear behaviour in total ankle replacement: a comparison between an in vitro simulation and retrieved prostheses. Clin Biomech 2009;24:661–9.
35. Karantana A, Hobson S, Dhar S. The Scandinavian total ankle replacement. Survivorship at 5 and 8 years comparable to other series. Clin Orthop Relat Res 2010;468:951–7.
36. Chou L, Coughlin M, Hansen S Jr, et al. Osteoarthritis of the ankle: the role of arthroplasty. J Am Acad Orthop Surg 2008;16:249–59.
37. Cracchiolo A, DeOrio J. Design features of current total ankle replacements: implants and instrumentation. J Am Acad Orthop Surg 2008;16:530–40.
38. DeOrio J, Easley M. Total ankle arthroplasty. AAOS Instr Course Lect 2008;57: 383–413.
39. Younger A, Penner M, Wing K. Mobile-bearing total ankle arthroplasty. Foot Ankle Clin 2008;13:495–508.
40. Shock RP, Christensen JC, Schuberth JM. Total ankle replacement in the varus ankle. J Foot Ankle Surg 2011;50(1):5–10.
41. Lee K, Lee Y, Young K, et al. Perioperative complications of the MOBILITY total ankle system: comparison with the HINTEGRA total ankle system. J Orthop Sci 2010;15:317–22.
42. Barg A, Elsner A, Hefti D, et al. Haemophilic arthropathy of the ankle treated by total ankle replacement: a case series. Haemophilia 2010;16:647–55.
43. Bai L, Lee K, Song E. Total ankle arthroplasty outcome comparison for post-traumatic and primary osteoarthritis. Foot Ankle Int 2010;31:1048–56.
44. Koivu H, Kohonen I, Sipola E, et al. Severe periprosthetic osteolytic lesions after the Ankle Evolutive System total ankle replacement. J Bone Joint Surg Br 2009; 91:907–14.
45. Wood P, Sutton C, Mishra V, et al. A randomized, controlled trial of two mobile-bearing total ankle replacements. J Bone Joint Surg Br 2009;91:69–74.
46. Kim B, Knupp M, Zwicky L, et al. Total ankle replacement in association with hindfoot fusion. Outcome and complications. J Bone Joint Surg Br 2010;92:1540–7.
47. Doets HC, Brand R, Nelissen RG. Total ankle arthroplasty in inflammatory joint disease with use of two mobile bearing designs. J Bone Joint Surg Am 2006; 88(6):1272–84.
48. San Giovanni T, Keblish D, Thomas W, et al. Eight-year results of a minimally constrained total ankle arthroplasty. Foot Ankle Int 2006;27(6):418–26.
49. Haddad S, Coetzee C, Estok R, et al. Intermediate and long-term outcomes of total ankle arthroplasty and ankle arthrodesis. J Bone Joint Surg Am 2007;89: 1899–905.

Subtalar Arthroereisis

Peter Highlander, DPM, MS[a], Wenjay Sung, DPM[b,*],
Lowell Weil Jr, DPM, MBA[c]

KEYWORDS

• Arthroereisis • Subtalar joint • Joint eversion • Implants

Arthroereisis is defined as an operative procedure with the goal of limiting a joint to a particular motion. Subtalar arthroereisis refers to the use of an implant positioned in the sinus tarsi and used as an endo-orthotic to limit excessive pronation of the subtalar joint (STJ). In turn this limitation prevents the sequela of overpronation while permitting inversion to occur unobstructed. The concept of subtalar arthroereisis was instituted in 1946 as Chambers[1] attempted to restrict STJ eversion through elevating the STJ posterior facet of the calcaneus at its anterior edge with bone graft. This altered the STJ axis of rotation and limited eversion. In 1952, Grice[2] reported his method of pediatric flatfoot reconstruction, using a cortical bone graft to hold the sinus tarsi open, creating an extra-articular subtalar arthrodesis; this procedure is no longer implemented, however, due to high incidence of degenerative arthritis.[2] Today, advances in techniques and materials continue, but subtalar arthroereisis remains controversial, especially in regards to indications, age at time of surgery, and adjunctive procedures.[3–6]

STJ arthroereisis has been advocated as an option for flexible flatfoot in children and adults. Flexible flatfoot is a common disorder and has a reported incidence of 5% in children and adults[7]; however, the true incidence is unknown. A flatfoot is characterized by plantar flexion and medial rotation of the talus, calcaneal eversion, medial longitudinal arch collapse, and abduction of the forefoot. Functionally, a flatfoot may be described as a foot that is undergoing pronation in the typical supinatory phases of gait or a foot that remains pronated during propulsion. The mass amount of structural (osseous) instability present is too much for the muscular and ligamentous structures to control. Over time, these soft tissues adapt by becoming more flexible and attenuated. The goal of arthroereisis is to limit overpronation, restoring normal anatomic relationships of the talocalcaneal and talonavicular joints. Subsequently, restoration of anatomic alignment reduces the forces on the surrounding soft tissues, including the long plantar ligament and plantar fascia. This allows the windlass mechanism to function and become more efficient in arch maintenance. Weight-bearing loads are shifted from the medial column to the lateral column; subluxation of medial joints is

[a] University of Pittsburgh Medical Center, Pittsburgh, PA, USA
[b] Sinai Medical Group, Department of Surgery, 1108 South Kedzie Avenue, Chicago, IL 60612, USA
[c] Weil Foot and Ankle Institute, 1455 East Golf Road, Des Plaines, IL 60016, USA
* Corresponding author.
E-mail address: wenjay.sung@sinai.org

Clin Podiatr Med Surg 28 (2011) 745–754
doi:10.1016/j.cpm.2011.08.004
0891-8422/11/$ – see front matter © 2011 Elsevier Inc. All rights reserved.

limited and pain reduced.[8] One theory by Roth and colleagues[9] states that with an arthroereisis implant in place, correction is achieved by stimulating the proprioceptive foot receptors, allowing active inversion but blocking excessive heel eversion. The permanence of correction is theoretically advantageous as well. When used in an immature skeleton, the bones may remodel in the corrected position, which is maintained once mature. According to Needleman,[10] for adults, an arthroereisis device in place for 8 months allows stiffening and remodeling of soft tissues, which are vital for joint alignment.

Arthroereisis has gained popularity over the years because it eliminates excessive pronation while conserving preoperative inversion and preserves forefoot to rearfoot adaptation to uneven terain.[11] Technically simple, some of the advantages of subtalar arthroereisis are that it is joint sparing and preserves ligaments. In addition, the implant does not interfere with osseous growth and does not compromise future operative intervention if more invasive procedures are required.[12] Arthroereisis, however, can have associated complications along with the need for surgical removal in some patient populations.

INDICATIONS AND CONTRAINDICATIONS

The primary indication for arthroereisis is for flexible flatfoot, also referred to as collapsing pes planovalgus. Collapsing refers to the flexibility of the arch and rearfoot structures to compensate for weight-bearing loads.[13] The development of a symptomatic flexible flatfoot is often bimodal. It may occur in adolescence and many times is idiopathic; later, in adults primarily in their fifth or sixth decade, the disorder is frequently acquired. Regardless of age, symptoms usually involve pain while walking or standing, postural fatigue, or cramping sensation in the foot or arch. Night cramps, lower back or knee pain, or sedentary preference may also be reasons for patients to seek medical intervention. Parents may state their child has as having a clumsy gait or preferring to be carried, or they may notice a decrease in activity.[14]

Pediatric flexible flatfoot rarely requires surgical intervention and represents normal pedal development for children under age 6 after which the deformity may correct itself with time.[15,16] Spontaneous correction is unlikely in children between 10 and 12 years old.[15,16] Often the pediatric flexible flatfoot is asymptomatic, and conservative measures, such as new footwear and orthotics, are indicated.[17] When a flexible flatfoot is symptomatic and conservative modalities have failed, surgical intervention is indicated. Arthroereisis may be considered in certain patients for operative management of pediatric symptomatic flexible flatfoot.[12] According to Koning and colleagues,[11] arthroereisis has little lasting effect beyond age 10 and the ideal age for arthroereisis for children is 8. Other investigators[18–20] have cautioned against early surgical intervention due to risk of development of cavovarus deformity, as observed by Villadot.[21]

Arthroereisis has also been shown beneficial for rigid flatfoot deformity resulting from tarsal coalition. Giannini and colleagues[18] reported good results in a series of pediatric patients with talocalcaneal coalition who were surgically managed with coalition resection and adjunctive bioabsorbable arthroereisis.

Relative contraindications for arthroereisis include angular deformity at the knee and torsional deformities. Caution should be used with arthroereisis in the presence of skew foot because the forefoot misalignment may be exacerbated if not addressed.[22] The stability of the midtarsal joint should also be evaluated preoperatively and intraoperatively. If instability exists at the midtarsal joint, an osteotomy may be indicated.[10] Absolute contraindications[22,23] include STJ arthritis, peroneal muscle spasm, and excessive ligamentous laxity, including generalized dysplasia.

TYPES OF IMPLANTS

A variety of arthroereisis implants are currently available. Vogler divided the implants into 3 categories based on biomechanical properties: axis altering, impact blocking, and self-locking.[24] Axis- altering implants create a more vertical STJ axis thus limiting frontal plane motion (eversion). Impact-blocking implants possess a platform and stem. The stem is inserted into the calcaneus just in front of the posterior STJ while the platform or cap projects superior, obstructing the lateral talar process excursion. The self-locking designed implants have a threaded portion, which is inserted into the sinus tarsi, thereby limiting talar plantarflexion and adduction while limiting calcaneal eversion. This style has many modifications and is the most common design used currently.

Some implants cross into several categories, but generally, implants can be divided into three groups: bioabsorbable, nonabsorbable, or combination. The vast majority of absorbable implants used currently are created from poly-L-lactic acid or ultrahigh molecular weight polyethylene. Bioabsorbable implants avoid the necessity of implant removal and sinus tarsi tenderness associated with prolonged placement of nonabsorbable implants; however, bioabsorbable implants are associated with additional complications. Giannini and colleagues[25] noted poly-L-lactic acid implants showed a loss of integrity after 1 year but results were good at 4-year follow-up.

In 1976, the Smith subtalar arthroereisis (STA-peg) implant (Wright Pharmaceutical, Arlington, TN, USA) was made of ultrahigh molecular weight polyethylene disk and stem and originally came in 2 sizes and was considered an axis-altering device according to Vogler's classification.[26] The STA-peg is traditionally placed in the floor of the sinus tarsi so the posterior facet of the talus can glide onto the dorsal surface of the implant, thereby preventing plantarflexion and medial rotation of the talus. The STA-peg was modified with an anterior incline to further increase the blockade and decrease medial rotation. Sgarlato Labs (Los Gatos, CA, USA) offers a similar design called the Lundeen Subtalar Implant, which has a longer stem and 5 sizes. This placement enabled the dorsal aspect of the disk to come in contact with the lateral leading wall of the talus. According to Forg and colleagues,[13] the Flake modification is useful in high STJ axis that is a largely transverse planar dominant flatfoot.

In addition to conventional screws, other nonabsorable arthroereisis implants are commonly used. The most common is the Maxwell-Brancheau Arthroereisis (MBA) (KMI, Carlsbad, CA, USA). The MBA is a self-locking titanium implant with a cannulated threaded cylinder and is slotted to allow soft tissue ingrowth, which helps anchor the implant.[22] This implant is inserted through the sinus tarsi and rests on the floor of the sinus tarsi (**Figs. 1** and **2**). The MBA implant is available in 5 sizes (6-mm, 8-mm, 9-mm, 10-mm, and 12-mm diameters). The range of sizes makes the MBA more versatile than traditional polyethylene implants.[23]

The Kalix endorthesis (Newdeal SA, Vienne, France) consists of a titanium cone trunk, which is inserted into another polyethylene cone trunk. According to Viladot and colleagues,[21] the Kalix endorthesis provides inherent advantages. The Kalix endorthesis had excellent results in biomechanical tests for compression and fatigue. Furthermore, the conical trunk shape adapts to the sinus tarsi shape better than cylindrical-shaped implants and the expansion mechanism and lateral fins prevent the implant from being displaced.[27] The Kalix endorthesis was approved by the Food and Drug Administration in 2000 and is available in the United States and Europe.

Other implants within the self-locking category are the Conical Subtalar Implant (CSI) (Nexa Orthopedics, San Diego, CA, USA), HyProCure (GraMedica, Macomb, MI, USA), Talar-Fit (OsteoMed, Dallas, TX, USA), and Talus of Vilex (TOV) (Vilex,

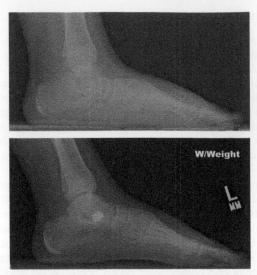

Fig. 1. Preoperative (*top*) and postoperative (*bottom*) lateral radiographs of a 9-year-old boy who underwent gastrocneumius recession and implantation of MBA arthroereisis for treatment of painful flexible pes planus. To date this patient has had no recurrence of symptoms and has not required any further surgical or nonsurgical care.

McMinnville, TN, USA). The CSI implant is titanium and is available in 6 sizes. The CSI was designed to enhance fit within the sinus tarsi; however, no published data are available to confirm this idea. The HyProCure implant is described as a "self-seating stent" by its manufacturer. Its unique design encompasses a distal threaded section, which allows tissue on-growth rather than engaging the walls of the sinus tarsi;

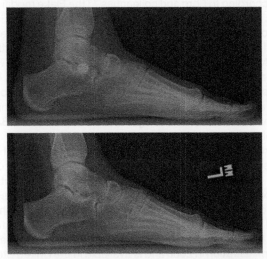

Fig. 2. Lateral radiographs of an 18-year-old woman who experienced unresolving sinus tarsi pain after insertion of an MBA subtalar arthroereisis several years before presentation (*top*). The implant was removed and symptoms were resolved with minimal loss of correction (*bottom*).

a central smooth tapered section, which allows equal pressure to be distributed and prevents over insertion; and a grooved head, which also permits tissue on-growth providing additional stability. The Talar-Fit implant possesses a conical shape and rounded deep treaded body and is available in 5 sizes. The titanium TOV implant is available in sizes 8 mm to 18 mm and is conical in shape (**Figs. 3** and **4**).

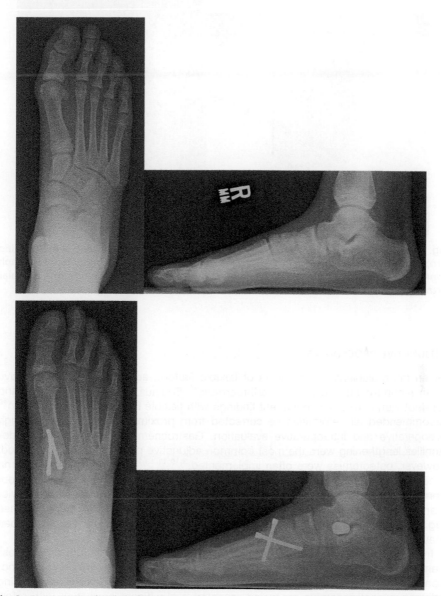

Fig. 3. Preoperative (*top*) and postoperative (*bottom*) radiographs of a 13-year-old girl with a 2 year history of painful hallux valgus and pes planus deformity. Patient underwent a gastrocnemius recession, Lapidus bunionectomy, and subtalar arthroereisis with the TOV implant without complication.

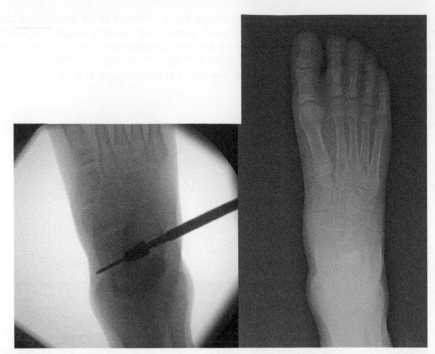

Fig. 4. Intraoperative radiograph (*left*) of an 11-year-old female patient demonstrating proper placement of a 10-mm TOV implant. Postoperative anteroposterior radiograph (*right*) of the same patient who underwent a Kidner procedure in addition to subtalar arthroereisis.

ADJUNCTIVE PROCEDURES

Given the multiplanar components of flexible flatfoot, adjunctive procedures have been recommended to subtalar arthroereisis.[10] Equinus, midtarsal instability, and forefoot varus are often concurrent findings with flexible flatfeet.[3,10,22] Needleman[10] recommended all deformities be corrected from proximal to distal with thorough preoperative and intraoperative evaluation. Gastrocnemius recession and tendo-Achilles lengthening were the most common adjunctive procedures recommended; however, osteotomies were often implemented.[3,10,11,13,19,21,25,28–30] Medial column reconstruction has been reported when forefoot varus is unmasked after flafoot correction.[3,10,13,30] A Kidner procedure may be appropriate when an accessory navicular is encountered to prevent recurrence or progression of the deformity (see **Fig. 4**).[3,10,13,30] Posterior tibial tendon insufficiency or spring ligament rupture repair may also be warranted in the acquired flatfoot population.[10,21,28]

In a case series of 20 pediatric patients (28 feet), Cicchinelli and colleagues[3] demonstrated significant correction when arthroereisis was performed in conjunction with gastrocnemius recession. When compared with arthroereisis alone, using adjunctive gastrocnemius recession revealed a significant correction with reference to talar axis and lesser tarsus axis angles.[3] They concluded, however, that an additional medial column reconstruction may limit correction given by the STJ implant.[3]

RESULTS

The extent of correction and biomechanical consequences of subtalar arthroereisis have been the topic of choice for multiple cadaveric and clinical studies. In two separate cadaveric reports, similar conclusions were made. Although the subtalar arthroereisis implant contacts the talus and calcaneus, the alignment of the remaining tarsal bones improved as well.[7,31] Christensen and colleagues[7] in a cadaveric study revealed the degree of change in talar position was similar in abduction and dorsiflexion. These findings indicated that there was no predilection for correction in the transverse and sagittal planes with arthroereisis. Other studies found similar results.[3,13,20,21,28,29] Husain and Fallat[23] quantified the degree of limited STJ range of motion based on size of MBA implants. They found that STJ range of motion was decreased by 32.0%, 44.8%, 58%, 65.5%, and 76.8% for 6-mm, 8-mm, 9-mm, 10-mm, and 12-mm implants, respectively.[23] They also believed that the consequences of altering STJ position from everted to inverted increased tension on the Achilles tendon; however, their observation was not quantified.[23]

The amount of correction provided by arthroereisis is difficult to quantify given the many adjunctive procedures performed; however, it seems that much of the correction is dependent on the magnitude of the deformity preoperatively and the size of the implant used. Reviewing case series data from the past decade reveals the principle correction occurs in the limitation of talar motion in the transverse and sagittal planes.[3,10,11,13,19–21,25,28,29] Subtalar arthroereisis may be used for flexible flatfoot reconstruction regardless of the dominant plane of deformity; however, it is difficult to assess frontal plane correction via plain film evaluation.[3]

Radiographic data and subjective results have been promising for both pediatrics and adults. Reviewing case series data within the past decade revealed a satisfaction rate ranging from 81% to 90% for pediatrics.[11,13,19] Satisfaction rates of 78% and 89% have been reported for adult patients.[10,21] Dramatic improvements in the American Orthopaedic Foot & Ankle Society (AOFAS) clinical rating system[32] have also been reported for children and adults. Giannini and colleagues[25] report an improvement of average AOFAS hindfoot scores from 29 preoperatively to 90 postoperatively in 12 patients who underwent tarsal coalition resection and subtalar arthroereisis. Other investigators[10,21] have reported final AOFAS hindfoot scores ranging from 82 to 90.

COMPLICATIONS

Despite good outcomes reported in the literature and ease of placement, subtalar arthroereisis can have associated complications. The majority of the complications are attributed to the implant itself causing discomfort or becoming dislocated (see **Fig. 2**; **Figs. 5** and **6**). For the pediatric population, complication rates of 15% and 29.6% have been reported.[11,20] Incidence of sinus tarsi pain has been reported as high as 46% in the adult population.[10] Much of the pain leads to surgical revision, including removal or relocation of the implant. The rate of implants requiring removal has been reported up to 39% in pediatric patients and even higher in adult patients.[10,13,20,21,25,28]

For these reasons, it is not uncommon for surgeons to routinely remove the implants.[11,19] Minimal loss of correction, however, can be expected if removal is indicated (see **Fig. 2**). In a prospective case report, Needleman[10] observed only a minimal loss of correction in patients in whom the implants were removed after 8 months.

Other complications that have been reported include foreign body synoviits[30] with extensive granulomatous giant cell reaction and bilateral intraossoeous cysts[33] in

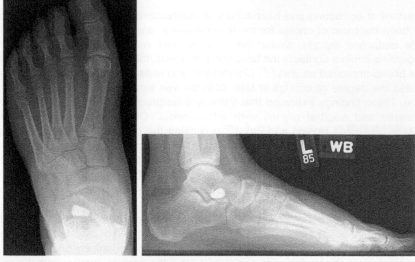

Fig. 5. Lateral radiograph demonstrates an anteriorly placed STJ implant, which caused pain. The implant was removed and symptoms resolved.

the talus. Siff and Granberry[34] reported a case of avascular necrosis of the talus associated with foreign body reaction to polyethylene debris 10 years after implantation. Additional complications reported include superficial wound infection[11] and peroneal spasm.[13] Undercorrection and overcorrection due to improper sizing of the implant have also been reported.[20]

FUTURE OUTLOOK

This report outlines use of subtalar arthroereisis for pediatric and adult acquired flexible flatfoot. Results obtained from the past decade are promising and similar to older studies[6,26,27,35] reported in the 1990s. Despite a high incidence of sinus tarsi pain, subtalar arthroereisis continues to be an alternative to joint destructive procedures. Although promising, there has only been one prospective study[10] and one study of pediatric patients, with follow-up averaging more than 12 years.[11] There is a need for higher level of evidence studies with long-term results to validate subtalar arthroereisis as a corrective procedure for flexible flatfoot.

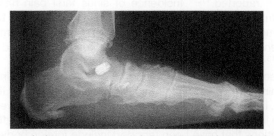

Fig. 6. Lateral radiograph demonstrating a dislocated STJ implant, which required removal.

REFERENCES

1. Chambers EF. An operation for the correction of flexible flat feet of adolescents. West J Surg Obstet Gynecol 1946;54:77.
2. Grice DS. An extra-articular arthrodesis of the subastragalar joint for correction of paralytic flat feet in children. J Bone Joint Surg Am 1952;34:927.
3. Cicchinelli LD, Pascual Huerta J, Garcia Carmona FJ, et al. Analysis of gastrocnemius recession and medial column procedures as adjuncts in arthroereisis for the correction of pediatric pes planovalgus: a radiographic retrospective study. J Foot Ankle Surg 2008;47:385.
4. Lepow GM, Smith SD. A modified subtalar arthroereisis implant for the correction of flexible flatfoot in children. The STA Peg procedure. Clin Podiatr Med Surg 1989;6:585.
5. Smith SD, Ocampo RF. Subtalar arthrorisis and associated procedures. Clin Podiatr Med Surg 1997;14:87.
6. Vedantam R, Capelli AM, Schoenecker PL. Subtalar arthroereisis for the correction of planovalgus foot in children with neuromuscular disorders. J Pediatr Orthop 1998;18:294.
7. Christensen JC, Campbell N, DiNucci K. Closed kinetic chain tarsal mechanics of subtalar joint arthroereisis. J Am Podiatr Med Assoc 1996;86:467.
8. Arangio GA, Reinert KL, Salathe EP. A biomechanical model of the effect of subtalar arthroereisis on the adult flexible flat foot. Clin Biomech (Bristol, Avon) 2004;19:847.
9. Roth S, Sestan B, Tudor A, et al. Minimally invasive calcaneo-stop method for idiopathic, flexible pes planovalgus in children. Foot Ankle Int 2007;28:991.
10. Needleman RL. A surgical approach for flexible flatfeet in adults including a subtalar arthroereisis with the MBA sinus tarsi implant. Foot Ankle Int 2006;27:9.
11. Koning PM, Heesterbeek PJ, de Visser E. Subtalar arthroereisis for pediatric flexible pes planovalgus: fifteen years experience with the cone-shaped implant. J Am Podiatr Med Assoc 2009;99:447.
12. Crawford AH, Kucharzyk D, Roy DR, et al. Subtalar stabilization of the planovalgus foot by staple arthroereisis in young children who have neuromuscular problems. J Bone Joint Surg Am 1990;72:840.
13. Forg P, Feldman K, Flake E, et al. Flake-Austin modification of the STA-Peg arthroereisis: a retrospective study. J Am Podiatr Med Assoc 2001;91:394.
14. Smith SD, Millar EA. Arthrorisis by means of a subtalar polyethylene peg implant for correction of hindfoot pronation in children. Clin Orthop Relat Res 1983;15.
15. Staheli LT, Chew DE, Corbett M. The longitudinal arch. A survey of eight hundred and eighty-two feet in normal children and adults. J Bone Joint Surg Am 1987; 69:426.
16. Welton EA. The Harris and Beath footprint: interpretation and clinical value. Foot Ankle 1992;13:462.
17. Soomekh DJ, Baravarian B. Pediatric and adult flatfoot reconstruction: subtalar arthroereisis versus realignment osteotomy surgical options. Clin Podiatr Med Surg 2006;23:695.
18. Giannini S, Ceccarelli F, Vannini F, et al. Operative treatment of flatfoot with talocalcaneal coalition. Clin Orthop Relat Res 2003;178.
19. Jerosch J, Schunck J, Abdel-Aziz H. The stop screw technique—a simple and reliable method in treating flexible flatfoot in children. Foot Ankle Surg 2009; 15:174.

20. Scharer BM, Black BE, Sockrider N. Treatment of painful pediatric flatfoot with Maxwell-Brancheau subtalar arthroereisis implant a retrospective radiographic review. Foot Ankle Spec 2010;3:67.
21. Viladot R, Pons M, Alvarez F, et al. Subtalar arthroereisis for posterior tibial tendon dysfunction: a preliminary report. Foot Ankle Int 2003;24:600.
22. Maxwell JR, Carro A, Sun C. Use of the Maxwell-Brancheau arthroereisis implant for the correction of posterior tibial tendon dysfunction. Clin Podiatr Med Surg 1999;16:479.
23. Husain ZS, Fallat LM. Biomechanical analysis of Maxwell-Brancheau arthroereisis implants. J Foot Ankle Surg 2002;41:352.
24. Banks AS, Downey MS, Martin DE, et al. McGlamry's comprehensive textbook of foot and ankle surgery. Philadelphia (PA): Lippincott Williams & Wilkins; 2001.
25. Giannini BS, Ceccarelli F, Benedetti MG, et al. Surgical treatment of flexible flatfoot in children a four-year follow-up study. J Bone Joint Surg Am 2001; 83(Suppl 2 Pt 2):73.
26. Pomeroy GC, Manoli A 2nd. A new operative approach for flatfoot secondary to posterior tibial tendon insufficiency: a preliminary report. Foot Ankle Int 1997; 18:206.
27. Chi TD, Toolan BC, Sangeorzan BJ, et al. The lateral column lengthening and medial column stabilization procedures. Clin Orthop Relat Res 1999;81.
28. Adelman VR, Szczepanski JA, Adelman RP. Radiographic evaluation of endo-scopic gastrocnemius recession, subtalar joint arthroereisis, and flexor tendon transfer for surgical correction of stage II posterior tibial tendon dysfunction: a pilot study. J Foot Ankle Surg 2008;47:400.
29. Nelson SC, Haycock DM, Little ER. Flexible flatfoot treatment with arthroereisis: radiographic improvement and child health survey analysis. J Foot Ankle Surg 2004;43:144.
30. Scher DM, Bansal M, Handler-Matasar S, et al. Extensive implant reaction in failed subtalar joint arthroereisis: report of two cases. HSS J 2007;3:177.
31. Giorgini RJ, Schiraldi FG, Hernandez PA. Subtalar arthroereisis: a combined technique. J Foot Surg 1988;27:157.
32. Kitaoka HB, Alexander IJ, Adelaar RS, et al. Clinical rating systems for the ankle-hindfoot, midfoot, hallux, and lesser toes. Foot Ankle Int 1994;15:349.
33. Rockett AK, Mangum G, Mendicino SS. Bilateral intraosseous cystic formation in the talus: a complication of subtalar arthroeresis. J Foot Ankle Surg 1998;37:421.
34. Siff TE, Granberry WM. Avascular necrosis of the talus following subtalar arthrori-sis with a polyethylene endoprosthesis: a case report. Foot Ankle Int 2000; 21:247.
35. Mosca VS. Calcaneal lengthening for valgus deformity of the hindfoot. Results in children who had severe, symptomatic flatfoot and skewfoot. J Bone Joint Surg Am 1995;77:500.

Total First Metatarsophalangeal Joint Implant Arthroplasty: A 30-year Retrospective

Wenjay Sung, DPM[a],*, Lowell Weil Jr, DPM, MBA[b],
Lowell Scott Weil Sr, DPM[b], Travis Stark, BS[b]

KEYWORDS

- First metatarsophalangeal joint • Arthroplasty • Implant

The first metatarsophalangeal (MTP) joint is the most frequent diseased-affected articulation encountered by the foot and ankle surgeon.[1,2] The standard initial treatment typically involves nonsteroidal anti-inflammatory medication, modification of shoes and activity, and orthotic inserts.[1] When these initial treatments fail to provide relief, surgical correction of the joint pathology is proposed.

Arthrodesis can be a satisfactory salvage operation,[3,4] but it must be done with precision, to place the great toe in the best position for each individual patient. First MTP joint arthrodesis has been reserved for patients who have an active lifestyle and engage in daily activities of high demand, such as heavy manual labor and sports.[5] Although joint arthrodesis has become the gold standard treatment for end-stage arthritis of this joint,[6,7] there are still complications associated with the procedure.[7]

Arthroplasty remains a favorable option for most surgeons, because it preserves motion of the joint. The first MTP joint resectional arthroplasty, described by Keller in 1904, proved to be a powerful surgical procedure to treat recalcitrant pain and end-stage arthritis of the first metatarsophalangeal joint.[8,9] However, the procedure has been associated with high complications rates and unpredictable results, especially in active adult patients.[10,11]

Trying to improve on the resectional arthroplasty, Swanson[12,13] introduced the single-stem silicone implant for first MTP joint hemi-arthroplasty, but his results

---

[a] Sinai Medical Group, Department of Surgery, 1108 South Kedzie Avenue, Chicago, IL 60612, USA
[b] Weil Foot and Ankle Institute, 1455 East Golf Road, Des Plaines, IL 60016, USA
* Corresponding author. Sinai Medical Group, 1108 South Kedzie Avenue, Chicago, IL 60612-3935.
E-mail address: wenjay.sung@sinai.org

Clin Podiatr Med Surg 28 (2011) 755–761
doi:10.1016/j.cpm.2011.08.005
0891-8422/11/$ – see front matter © 2011 Elsevier Inc. All rights reserved.

podiatric.theclinics.com

continued to be less than satisfactory. The double-stem silicone implants for total joint arthroplasty[1,14,15] were the next step in implant evolution. Cook and colleagues[14] outlined this evolution of first MTP implant material and designs. Although there appear to be f4 generations of total first MTP implants, most of the collected data for long-term studies have been focused on the silicone implant generation.

The mechanical demands, biomechanical complexity, and material interactions relating to the first MTP joint have influenced designs and materials.[16–18] Various biomaterials have been employed as joint spacers or functional implants to replace the diseased or resected segment of bone.[19] The consensus within the literature has expressed optimism regarding the recent generation of total joint implants; however, many continue to believe that there is a lack of satisfactory results regarding the functional outcomes of total joint implant.[14] However, patient satisfaction with total first MTP joint implant arthroplasty remains high when compared with other joint replacements.[20–22]

As innovative materials and designs continue to improve, future studies on the newer generation of total first MTP joint implants will become available. The authors' focus at the Weil Foot and Ankle Institute has been on using double-stem silicone implants with titanium grommets,[23,24] and they believe it is a viable solution for affected articulations. The authors present their clinical results from over 30 years of experience with total first MTP joint implant arthroplasty at the Weil Foot and Ankle Institute.

SURGICAL CONSIDERATIONS

By definition, implant arthroplasty is a joint destructive procedure used in situations where integrity of joint is lost beyond intrinsic anatomic reconstruction.[25,26] Implant arthroplasty serves as an alternative solution for a patient in whom joint arthrodesis, metatarsal osteotomy, or excisional type arthroplasty may not be ideal. Identifying this patient subtype and the different styles of specific implants are what troubles most surgeons in recognizing this as a consistent treatment option.[25]

The first MTP total joint implant can be classified most simply on the basis of being interpositional or joint replacement. It is very important to consider the type of implant and its material. Ideal implant properties are inert, nonbiodegradable, durable, nonirritating devices that recreate or enhance motion about the first MTP joint. These biomaterials can consist of ceramic, polyethylene, silicone rubber, stainless steel, cobalt chromium alloy, or titanium alloy. Composites such as steel and polyethylene, plasma-sprayed titanium, or hydroxyapetite have become popular implant materials in recent years. These materials can be manufactured for biologic ingrowths, mechanical interlock, press fit, screw fixation, or cementing.

The primary indications for first MTP joint implants are hallux rigidus, hallux valgus, rheumatoid arthritic joint, failure of previous operations, osteoarthritis, gouty arthritis, and Reiter syndrome.[1,7,27–30] A main goal for any total joint arthroplasty is to relieve pain, provide adequate range of motion, offer mechanical advantage and stability, and preserve cosmetic appearance by restoring adequate length.[28] First MTP joint implant arthroplasty indications are not specific to disease, but also the functional demands anticipated by the patient after surgical intervention. Total implant arthroplasty finds its primary use in situations where excisional arthroplasty or arthrodesis may also be indicated, but its advantages are in patients seeking to preserve or enhance motion.[1] In the authors' experience, the female population may resist first MTP arthrodesis more than males. Socioeconomic status and population density also play roles in patient resistance, as patients may wish to maintain range of motion of the joint to wear fashionable shoes. However, it is imperative that the surgeon carefully decides with the patient the correct procedure, and that the decision is not one-sided toward either party.

Absolute contraindications are joint infection, wound healing deficiencies, and allergy to implant materials. Active and functionally demanding lifestyle remains a relative contraindication. There is evidence that shows patients who are significantly younger are predisposed toward implant failure.[14,31]

MATERIALS AND METHODS

The authors reviewed medical records of consecutive adult patients who underwent a total first MTP joint implant arthroplasty from January 1979 until December 2002 at the Weil Foot and Ankle Institute. This included outpatient clinical office notes and hospital records. Medical records were sorted by hand or reviewed by electronic medical record. Patient medical records were only included in this review if there were attached radiographs depicting preoperative pathology and postoperative results from anterior–posterior and lateral views. After review, 283 patients who had undergone total first MTP joint implant arthroplasty had complete medical records. The authors then thoroughly reviewed the data to only include patients who had at least 24 months of follow-up after surgery. In total, there were 69 patients (92 feet) who formed the basis for this review.

The surgical technique was a modification from Swanson and de Groot Swanson.[23] This consisted of a dorsomedial incision along the first MTP joint. Once the joint was exposed, the cartilage and subchondral plate were removed from the first metatarsal head and base of the proximal phalanx. A large McGlamry elevator released the inferior attachments to the base of the metatarsal head. The proximal phalanx was aligned with the first metatarsal to reveal any abductus or angular deformity. An oscillating saw was used to make perpedicular cuts 0.5 cm from the edge of the metatarsal head and base of the proximal phalanx. Increased abductus was corrected with the oscillating saw cuts. The authors use a 90° bone clamp to retract the proximal phalanx by wrapping around the phalanx cortex beneath the soft tissue. While distracting the phalanx, the large McGlamry elevator can be positioned inferior to the metatarsal while a thin burr is used to core out 1 cm of meduallary bone from the dorsal center of the shaft. An implant trochar is used to fashion the proper size for the proximal stem of the implant. A similar procedure is then also done to the proximal phalanx shaft. Once a trial implant sizer with titanium grommets is applied into the fashioned space, the burr is used to remove prominent edges around the first MTP joint. After removal of the trial implant sizer, copious irrigation is applied to the first MTP joint. The titanium grommets with the silicone implant are then introduced into the joint and press-fitted. Range of motion is tested, and if satisfactory, closure of capsule and skin can proceed. All skin sutures are dissolvable and intercuticularly closed.

All patients were weight-bearing as tolerated without assistance the day of surgery. Their sterile compressive dressings were to remain clean, dry, and intact until the week after surgery. One week after surgery, all dressings were removed, and patients were allowed to return into comfortable, spacious shoes. Follow-up intervals were routinuely 1, 3, 6, 12, and 24 weeks postoperatively. All patients in this review had follow-up intervals greater than 24 months postoperatively.

Radiographic and clinically corresponding medical reports were used to determine stage of osteoarthritis preoperatively, if applicable. Complications in the perioperative period (3 months) included wound dehiscence, infection, implant rejection or failure, instability or malalignment, neuritis, and severe uncontrollable pain. Radiographic images and clinically corresponding medical reports postoperatively were evaluated to determine any implant fracture, malalignment after the initial postoperative period, implant failure, surgical revision, infection, and amputation.

Patients were asked to fill out the American Orthopaedic Foot and Ankle Society Hallux-Metatarsophalangeal Interphalangeal Scale[32] (AOFAS HMIS). A successful outcome was defined as achieving complete relief and satisfaction regarding their chief complaint after 24 months of postoperative follow-up.

RESULTS

The average age of the patients was 58.8 years (range 29–75 years) at time of operation and 66.0 (range 34–86 years) at time of last follow-up visit. Of the 63 patients, 6 were men, and 57 were women, and of the 92 feet included, there were 50 right feet, compared with 42 left feet. The average interval follow-up after surgery for all 63 patients was 86.7 months (range 24.5–333.9 months).

There were 19 patients who had previous surgery to the first MTP joint, 18 patients who were also treated for concurrent hallux valgus, 15 patients with tobacco history, 12 patients with diabetes mellitus with or without neuropathy, 10 patients with kidney disease, 6 patients with a history of rheumatoid arthritis, 3 patients with scleroderma, 2 patients with painful calluses, and 2 patients with a history of ulceration to the first ray. The average number of procedures performed concurrently with the total first MTP joint implant arthroplasty was 2.5 (range 1–7 concurrent procedures).

The average AOFAS HMIS was 82.4 (range 55–100) with a standard deviation (STDEV) of 12.0 (95% confidence interval of 78.8–86.0). Total range of motion was recorded postoperatively at final follow-up for an average of 56.6° (45.6° of dorsiflexion and 10.0° of plantarflexion). Complications in the postoperative period were found in 10 cases (10.4%). This included 5 ulcerations, 3 unresolved neuritis, and 2 incisional dehiscence complications. There were 13 cases (14.1%) of surgical revision at an average of 5.1 years (range 1–10 years) after surgery. Nine cases (9.8%) involved worn or failed implants that were replaced. There were 4 cases (4.3%) where the implant was removed. Of those 4 implant removals, two (2.2%) required amputation of the first ray. The authors' success rate was determined to be 85.9% in this series.

DISCUSSION

The authors believe that it is imperative to consider the individual requirements of a patient to select the proper procedure for first MTP pathology. As previously stated, the authors' success rate was 85.9% in this series, with 10.4% of cases that developed perioperative complications. This is similar to other authors[1,13,18,27–30,33–35] who have previously reported successful results using total first MTP implants to treat first MTP pathology, and in particular, using double-stem silicone implants with titanium grommets.[23,24,36]

Swanson has been credited with advancing total first MTP implant arthroplasty as a validated, successful alternative to arthrodesis.[12,15,30] His research is also known among hand surgeons for the successful treatments he developed in the upper extremity.[21,22] Since his research into total first MTP implant arthroplasties, many different implants have emerged with similar successful results. Cook and colleagues[14] have already complied and analyzed higher quality studies using meta-analysis techniques. The authors concluded that patient satisfaction was found to be 85.7% among all studies and 94.5% among higher-quality studies.[14] This is similar to the current authors' results.

Although Deheer has argued against the use of implant arthroplasties for the first MTP joint, his concerns focus on comparisons to results of first MTP arthrodesis.[25]

However, when compared with other implant arthroplasties in the body, total first MTP implant arthroplasty is similar if not more successful in clinical outcomes.[20–22] Coughlin recently touted that the evolution of implant arthroplasty versus arthrodesis has existed for many parts of the body.[37] Preferred treatment in orthopedics has shifted from repair to replace starting with the hip from the 1970s and the knee from the 1980s. However, only when arthroplasty has superior and consistent results when compared with fusion does the standard of care change. Until then, total implant arthroplasty for the first MTP joint will continue to be considered radical.

Reported complications to total first MTP implant arthroplasty vary with different studies, and many authors have used this inconsistency as validation for discouraging implant arthroplasties. Vanore and colleagues[38] reported silicone-induced synovitis, while Lim and colleagues[39] reported lymphadenopathy due to implant deterioration. Although Granberry and colleagues[27] reported high patient satisfaction rates, the authors noted the fracturing and destruction of the implant after long-term radiographic follow-up. However, Papagelopoulos and colleagues[31] studied long-term survival rate for total implant arthroplasties and concluded that survivorship of the implant in situ was 82% at 15 years after surgery. Furthermore, Mondul and colleagues[29] noted the disconnect between patient satisfaction, due to pain relief and cosmetic appearance, and radiographic changes. Callosities have also been noted to persist after implant arthroplasty.[27] Other complications include infection, wound dehiscence, and metatarsal fractures.

FUTURE OUTLOOK

The authors believe that their experience with total first MTP implant arthroplasty will add to the body of evidence in support for joint arthroplasty procedures. Although they provide level 4 evidence-based medicine with this retrospective cases series, the authors' results demonstrate that using double-stem silicone implants with titanium grommets for joint arthroplasty is a safe and effective treatment option for first MTP pathology.

REFERENCES

1. Cracchiolo A 3rd, Weltmer JB Jr, Lian G, et al. Arthroplasty of the first metatarsophalangeal joint with a double-stem silicone implant. Results in patients who have degenerative joint disease failure of previous operations or rheumatoid arthritis. J Bone Joint Surg Am 1992;74:552.
2. Muehleman C, Bareither D, Huch K, et al. Prevalence of degenerative morphological changes in the joints of the lower extremity. Osteoarthritis Cartilage 1997;5:23.
3. Coughlin MJ, Grebing BR, Jones CP. Arthrodesis of the first metatarsophalangeal joint for idiopathic hallux valgus: intermediate results. Foot Ankle Int 2005;26:783.
4. McKeever DC. Arthrodesis of the first metatarsophalangeal joint for hallux valgus, hallux rigidus, and metatarsus primus varus. J Bone Joint Surg Am 1952;34:129.
5. Pulavarti RS, McVie JL, Tulloch CJ. First metatarsophalangeal joint replacement using the bio-action great toe implant: intermediate results. Foot Ankle Int 2005;26:1033.
6. Brage ME, Ball ST. Surgical options for salvage of end-stage hallux rigidus. Foot Ankle Clin 2002;7:49.
7. Shereff MJ, Baumhauer JF. Hallux rigidus and osteoarthrosis of the first metatarsophalangeal joint. J Bone Joint Surg Am 1998;80:898.

8. Cleveland M, Winant EM. An end-result study of the Keller operation. J Bone Joint Surg Am 1950;32:163.

9. Keller W. Surgical treatment of bunions and hallux valgus. NY Med J 1904;80:741.

10. Vallier GT, Petersen SA, LaGrone MO. The Keller resection arthroplasty: a 13-year experience. Foot Ankle 1991;11:187.

11. Wrighton J. A ten-year review of Keller's operation. Clin Orthop 1972;89:207.

12. Swanson AB. Implant arthroplasty for the great toe. Clin Orthop Relat Res 1972; 85:75.

13. Swanson AB, Lumsden RM, Swanson GD. Silicone implant arthroplasty of the great toe. A review of single stem and flexible hinge implants. Clin Orthop Relat Res 1979;(142):30–43.

14. Cook E, Cook J, Rosenblum B, et al. Meta-analysis of first metatarsophalangeal joint implant arthroplasty. J Foot Ankle Surg 2009;48:180.

15. Cracchiolo A 3rd, Swanson A, Swanson GD. The arthritic great toe metatarsophalangeal joint: a review of flexible silicone implant arthroplasty from two medical centers. Clin Orthop Relat Res 1981;(157):64–9.

16. Merkle PF, Sculco TP. Prosthetic replacement of the first metatarsophalangeal joint. Foot Ankle 1989;9:267.

17. Seeburger RH. Surgical implants of alloyed metal in joints of the feet. J Am Podiatry Assoc 1964;54:391.

18. Sgarlato TE. Sutter double-stem silicone implant arthroplasty of the lesser metatarsophalangeal joints. J Foot Surg 1989;28:410.

19. Broughton NS, Doran A, Meggitt BF. Silastic ball spacer arthroplasty in the management of hallux valgus and hallux rigidus. Foot Ankle 1989;10:61.

20. Bullens PH, van Loon CJ, de Waal Malefijt MC, et al. Patient satisfaction after total knee arthroplasty: a comparison between subjective and objective outcome assessments. J Arthroplasty 2001;16:740.

21. Kimball HL, Terrono AL, Feldon P, et al. Metacarpophalangeal joint arthroplasty in rheumatoid arthritis. Instr Course Lect 2003;52:163.

22. Swanson AB, de Groot Swanson G, Ishikawa H. Use of grommets for flexible implant resection arthroplasty of the metacarpophalangeal joint. Clin Orthop Relat Res 1997;(342):22–33.

23. Swanson AB, de Groot Swanson G. Use of grommets for flexible hinge implant arthroplasty of the great toe. Clin Orthop Relat Res 1997;(340):87–94.

24. Swanson AB, de Groot Swanson G, Maupin BK, et al. The use of a grommet bone liner for flexible hinge implant arthroplasty of the great toe. Foot Ankle 1991;12:149.

25. Deheer PA. The case against first metatarsal phalangeal joint implant arthroplasty. Clin Podiatr Med Surg 2006;23:709.

26. Hanft JR, Merrill T, Marcinko DE, et al. Grand rounds: first metatarsophalangeal joint replacement. J Foot Ankle Surg 1996;35:78.

27. Granberry WM, Noble PC, Bishop JO, et al. Use of a hinged silicone prosthesis for replacement arthroplasty of the first metatarsophalangeal joint. J Bone Joint Surg Am 1991;73:1453.

28. Lemon B, Pupp GR. Long-term efficacy of total SILASTIC implants: a subjective analysis. J Foot Ankle Surg 1997;36:341.

29. Mondul M, Jacobs PM, Caneva RG, et al. Implant arthroplasty of the first metatarsophalangeal joint: a 12-year retrospective study. J Foot Surg 1985; 24:275.

30. Weil LS, Pollak RA, Goller WL. Total first joint replacement in hallux valgus and hallux rigidus. Long-term results in 484 cases. Clin Podiatry 1984;1:103.

31. Papagelopoulos PJ, Kitaoka HB, Ilstrup DM. Survivorship analysis of implant arthroplasty for the first metatarsophalangeal joint. Clin Orthop Relat Res 1994;(302):164–72.
32. Kitaoka HB, Alexander IJ, Adelaar RS, et al. Clinical rating systems for the ankle-hindfoot, midfoot, hallux, and lesser toes. Foot Ankle Int 1994;15:349.
33. Gerbert J, Chang TJ. Clinical experience with two-component first metatarsal phalangeal joint implants. Clin Podiatr Med Surg 1995;12:403.
34. Kampner SL. Total joint prosthetic arthroplasty of the great toe–a 12-year experience. Foot Ankle 1984;4:249.
35. Laird L. Silastic joint arthroplasty of the great toe. A review of 228 implants using the double-stemmed implant. Clin Orthop Relat Res 1990;(255):268–72.
36. Sebold EJ, Cracchiolo A 3rd. Use of titanium grommets in silicone implant arthroplasty of the hallux metatarsophalangeal joint. Foot Ankle Int 1996;17:145.
37. Coughlin M. Total ankle replacement: top 10 questions. In: Conference Proceedings of the New York Foot and Ankle Symposium. The Palace Hotel: New York, New York; 2010.
38. Vanore J, O'Keefe R, Pikscher I. Silastic implant arthroplasty. Complications and their classification. J Am Podiatry Assoc 1984;74:423.
39. Lim WT, Landrum K, Weinberger B. Silicone lymphadenitis secondary to implant degeneration. J Foot Surg 1983;22:243.

Current Concepts and Techniques
in Foot and Ankle Surgery

Transcalcaneal Talonavicular Dislocation Associated with an Open Comminuted Calcaneal Fracture: A Case Report

Spyridon P. Galanakos, MD, PhD*, Vassilios Papathanasiou, MD,
Ioannis P. Sofianos, MD

KEYWORDS

- Foot • Trauma • Dislocation • Open fracture
- Talus • Calcaneus

The combination of dorsal dislocation of the navicular from the talus and a comminuted fracture of the calcaneus (transcalcaneal talonavicular dislocation) is an unusual and severe injury.[1-3] It occurs due to a forced plantarflexion of the talar head through the anterior portion of the calcaneum and is usually associated with a potential for skin and neurovascular compromise. To the authors' knowledge, few cases have been reported previously in the literature.[1,3-5] This article reports an unusual case of an open transcalcaneal talonavicular dislocation associated with the presence of a calcaneal comminuted calcaneal fracture.

CASE REPORT

A 27-year-old healthy man, a manual worker, injured his left hindfoot after a fall from height while at work. After assessment in an accident and emergency department, he was found to have a deformity of his hindfoot and a wound measuring approximately 15 cm long extended from the medial malleolus to the plantar aspect of his heel with small bone fragments exposed in the wound. There was no neurovascular compromise in his injured left foot. Clinical photographs of the wound were taken, the wound

Conflict of interest: None of the authors of this manuscript has financial or personal relationships that could inappropriately influence the authors' decisions, work, or manuscript.
Department of Orthopaedics, General Hospital of Levadia, Levadia, Greece
* Corresponding author. 14-16 Trikalon Street, 11526, Ambelokipi, Athens, Greece.
E-mail address: Spyros_galanakos@yahoo.gr

Clin Podiatr Med Surg 28 (2011) 763–767
doi:10.1016/j.cpm.2011.07.002
0891-8422/11/$ – see front matter © 2011 Elsevier Inc. All rights reserved.

podiatric.theclinics.com

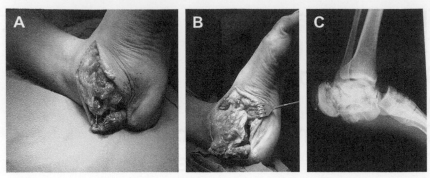

Fig. 1. Intraoperative appearance of the open calcaneal fracture (*A, B*) and lateral radiograph of the left foot and ankle showing the transcalcaneal talonavicular dislocation with an associated comminuted calcaneal fracture (*C*).

was covered with sterile dressing, adequate tetanus and antibiotic prophylaxis were administrated, and the foot was secured with a posterior fiberglass splint dressing (**Fig. 1**A, B).

Anteroposterior, lateral, and oblique radiographs of the foot and ankle were obtained and revealed a multifragmentary fracture of the calcaneum associated with a talonavicular dislocation. The talus was planterflexed with its head portion displaced plantarwards through the calcaneal fracture (see **Fig. 1**C). The radiologic findings revealed no other associated fractures.

The patient was brought to the operating room on an urgent basis and after induction of general anesthesia and sterile prepping, the wound was adequately excised to healthy margins and irrigated with at least 10 L of normal saline solution while the foot dislocation was reduced under C-arm fluoroscopy. The talonavicular joint was stabilized with 2-mm Kirschner wires (K-wires) introduced from the dorsal and medial aspect of the foot transfixing the talonavicular joint. Furthermore, the calcaneal fracture was manipulated through the open wound to obtain better alignment and using a hybrid Ace-Fisher External Fixation System (DePuy Ace, Warsaw, IN, USA). The reduction of the dislocation was achieved with satisfactory results and the foot and ankle were stabilized with the external fixation system. The traumatic wound was also closed primarily (**Fig. 2**).

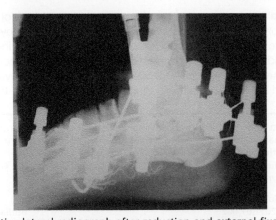

Fig. 2. Postoperative lateral radiograph after reduction and external fixator placement.

Intravenous antibiotics were continued 72 hours after the surgery and low molecular weight heparin prophylaxis was administered during the hospital course. Five days after the procedure, a minor surgical wound edge necrosis with superficial infection was developed and successfully treated with multiple operative irrigations, débridements, and oral antibiotics (**Fig. 3A**). The patient was discharged from the hospital on the twelfth postoperative day. Three weeks later, the wound was healed completely without any further complications and after that it was managed with normal dry sterile dressing changes (see **Fig. 3B**).

At 6 weeks postoperatively, the K-wires from the talonavicular joint were removed, but the hybrid fixator remained for an additional 10 weeks. The patient was to remain non–weight bearing for approximately 16 weeks. After the external fixator removal, the patient was allowed to maintain a weight-bearing status as tolerated with assistance of crutches. At the 8-month follow-up, he was able to walk with full weight bearing independently and the patient returned to his occupation as a clerk.

At the end of the first postoperative year, range of motion of his left ankle was dorsiflexion 5°, plantarflexion 40°, inversion 20°, and eversion 10°. Radiographs at that time showed mild degenerative changes at the talotibial joint and some degree of space narrowing at talotibial, talonavicular, and subtalar joints (**Fig. 4**). The American Orthopaedic Foot and Ankle Society hindfoot score[6] at 18 months was 63. After 2 years of the injury, the patient was lost to follow-up. No clinical or radiologic signs of osteomyelitis or avascular necrosis were developed until the last assessment.

DISCUSSION

Association of dorsal dislocation of the navicular from the talus with an open fracture of the calcaneus is an uncommon but severe injury. Coltart in 1952[1] was the first to report such injuries; he described 5 cases of severe comminution of the calcaneum with fracture through the neck of the talus with the body of the talus inverted and embedded in the calcaneum. He impressed that these injuries were severe and usually open and often became infected. Three of the 5 patients required a below-the-knee amputation. Kleiger[3] schematically described a similar type of injury with plantar dislocation of the talus at the talonavicular joint and calcaneal fracture as one of the mechanisms of talar injury. In 1993, Ebraheim and colleagues[2] reported two cases of complex fracture-dislocation of the calcaneus. A different mechanism of injury, from that in our study, was described, where the talus was dislocated and plantarflexed and the calcaneus was dislocated laterally with a highly comminuted fracture.

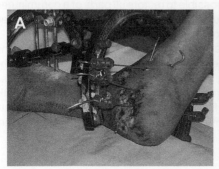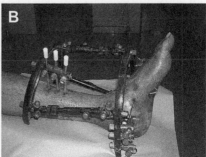

Fig. 3. A minor surgical wound edge necrosis with superficial infection was noted 5 days postoperatively (*A*) and clinical appearance of the foot and ankle with the apparatus at the fifth postoperative week (*B*).

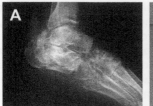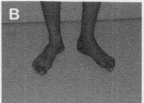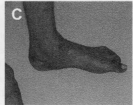

Fig. 4. Final radiograph (*A*) and clinical appearance of the left foot and ankle (*B, C*) at the end of the first postoperative year.

In addition, Ricci and colleagues[4] reported a detailed description of the transcalcaneal talonavicular dislocation and its variations in injury pattern with methods and treatment options. There were 9 cases of transcalcaneal talonavicular dislocation of which 5 were open injuries. Four of these developed osteomyelitis and 3 subsequently required amputation.

Open fractures of the calcaneum are rare injuries, representing between 0.8% and 10% of all os calcis fractures in published series.[7,8] Open calcaneal fractures are characterized by an increased frequency of infection despite the strict protocols of treating these complex open injuries. Associated complications may include but are not limited to sympathetic algodystrophy, subtalar arthritis, calcaneocuboid arthritis, malunion, tendinitis of fibularis, and remaining ankle pain.[9,10] No other major complications were noted in the authors' case patient.

It is known that the goals of open calcaneal fracture management include timely healing of the soft tissue without infection and maintenance of bony alignment.[11] Some investigators recommended that management of the soft tissue disruption and avoidance of infection should be the initial treatment focus rather than fracture stabilization.[10,12] The stability provided by early internal fixation of open fractures is believed, however, to diminish the risk of infection and promote healing of the injured soft tissues.[13,14] The characteristic of the authors' case patient's injury pattern was plantar dislocation of the talus from the navicular associated with a severely comminuted open calcaneal fracture. A remarkable functional outcome was achieved with one major surgical procedure, and only local further débridements were necessary due to minor wound problems.

Although general treatment recommendation for severely intra-articular fractures of the posterior facet is early or late subtalar arthrodesis,[11] immediate minimally invasive fixation with percutaneous pinning and external fixation needs to be considered for the healthy and active patients. It is usually not possible to restore all parts of a comminuted calcaneal fracture with an external fixator, but the aim of the apparatus in the presented case was to provide further stabilization and better alignment of the calcaneus.

In the authors' case report, the patient was able to walk with full weight bearing and without any assistance at the eighth postoperative month and he was pleased with the outcome. Posttraumatic arthritis, however, is usually a late phenomenon with these types of injuries and may need to be addressed if a patient becomes symptomatic in the future. The authors' percutaneous fixation technique was used to eliminate the option of a primary arthrodesis at the time of his severe open injury and significant amount of soft tissue loss.

SUMMARY

This article presents a case report of a plantar dislocation of the talus from the navicular associated with a severely comminuted open calcaneal fracture, managed by one surgical procedure and a good clinical outcome. Besides the good results of the case patient, the prognosis for most of these types of injuries varies from severe functional limitations and/or chronic pain to even amputation.

REFERENCES

1. Coltart WD. Aviator's astragalus. J Bone Joint Surg Br 1952;34:545–66.
2. Ebraheim NA, Savolaine ER, Paley K, et al. Comminuted fracture of the calcaneus associated with subluxation of the talus. Foot Ankle 1993;14:380–4.
3. Kleiger B. Injuries of the talus and its joints. Clin Orthop Relat Res 1976;121: 243–62.
4. Ricci WM, Bellabarba C, Sanders R. Transcalcaneal talonavicular dislocation. J Bone Joint Surg Am 2002;84:557–61.
5. Kamath RP, Chandran P, Nihal A. Transcalcaneal talonavicular dislocation. Foot Ankle Surg 2007;13:147–9.
6. Kitaoka HB, Alexander IJ, Adelaar RS, et al. Clinical rating systems for the ankle—hindfoot, midfoot, hallux and lesser toes. Foot Ankle Int 1994;15:349–53.
7. Benirschke SK, Sangeorzan BJ. Extensive intra-articular fractures of the foot. Clin Orthop Relat Res 1993;292:128–34.
8. Soeur R, Remy R. Fractures of the calcaneus with displacement of the thalamic portion. J Bone Joint Surg Br 1975;57:413–21.
9. Berry GK, Stevens DG, Kreder HJ, et al. Open fractures of the calcaneus. A review of treatment and outcome. J Orthop Trauma 2004;18:202–6.
10. Siebert CH, Hansen M, Wolter D. Follow-up evaluation of open intra-articular fractures of the calcaneus. Arch Orthop Trauma Surg 1998;117:442–7.
11. Lawrence SJ. Open calcaneal fractures. Orthopedics 2004;27(7):737–42.
12. Aldridge JM III, Easley M, Nunley JA. Open calcaneal fractures. J Orthop Trauma 2004;18:7–11.
13. Chapman MW, Mahoney M. The role of early internal fixation in the management of open fractures. Clin Orthop Relat Res 1979;138:120–31.
14. Franklin JL, Johnson KD, Hansen ST. Immediate internal fixation of open ankle fractures. Report of 38 cases treated with a standard protocol. J Bone Joint Surg Am 1984;66:1349–56.

Digital Arthrodesis: Current Fixation Techniques

Jared L. Moon, DPM[a],*, Carl A. Kihm, DPM[a], Daniel A. Perez, DPM[a],
Leslie B. Dowling, DPM, MBA[a], David C. Alder, DPM[a],[b]

KEYWORDS

• Proximal interphalangeal joint arthrodesis • Hammertoe
• Digital arthrodesis

Surgical correction of the hammertoe deformity often involves arthrodesis of the proximal interphalangeal joint (PIPJ). Glissan's principles must be appreciated for digital joint fusion regardless of how joint stability is achieved.[1] Traditional methods such as Kirschner-wire (K-wire) fixation are time-honored and remain an effective option; however, multiple new designs have been introduced in an attempt to provide more optimal fixation. Foot and ankle surgeons may now choose from the following implants: Smart Toe, HammerLock, Arrow-Lok, Pro-Toe VO, StayFuse, and cannulated screws. This article reviews these recently introduced digital implants in addition to more traditional fixation options for digital arthrodesis.

SMART TOE

The Smart Toe (MMI, Memometal, Inc, Memphis, TN, USA) digital implant is a one-piece system composed of NiTinol (Nickel Titanium Naval Ordinance Laboratory). NiTinol is an inert binary metal alloy consisting of approximately 50% nickel and 50% titanium.[2] This composition affords the implant the unique properties of "warm-shape" metal memory. Metal memory is acquired during the extensive manufacturing process of metal forging, lamination, wiredrawing, cutting, alloy education, folding, and buffing.[3] The implant is initially shaped and bent, and then returns to its original shape once heated past its transition temperature. The Smart Toe implant is maintained at less than 0°C for at least 2 hours before insertion. Shape recovery is initiated by the patient's body temperature on implant insertion. Once removed from the freezer, the surgeon has approximately 1.5 to 2 minutes of "work time" before expansion.[3] Care is taken not to touch the metal, as the surgeon's body heat will cause an immature expansion of the implant. The Smart Toe's metal memory properties have

The authors have nothing to disclose.
[a] DeKalb Medical Center, 2701 North Decatur Road, Decatur, GA 30033, USA
[b] Podiatry Institute, 2675 North Decatur Road, Street 309, Decatur, GA 30033, USA
* Corresponding author.
E-mail address: Jared.L.Moon@gmail.com

doi:10.1016/j.cpm.2011.07.003
0891-8422/11/$ – see front matter © 2011 Elsevier Inc. All rights reserved.
podiatric.theclinics.com

been incorporated into the design specifically to help compress the arthrodesis site and engage the internal bone cortices. As it is heated the implant returns to its original shape, causing it to expand in width as it shortens in length.

The implant is available in lengths of 16 or 19 mm, and can be either straight or plantarflexed at 10° to give the digit a more anatomic appearance. The implant is divided into proximal and distal portions that correspond to the regions inserted in the proximal and middle phalanx. The proximal portion ranges in width from 2.0 to 5.5 mm and the distal portion ranges from 3 to 6 mm. The length of the proximal portion is 10 mm for a 16-mm long implant and 13 mm for a 19-mm long implant. The proximal portion makes up approximately two-thirds of the implant length. All Smart Toe implants are 1.2 mm in thickness (**Fig. 1**).

Implant insertion is performed once the joint is properly resected. The intramedullary canals of both the middle and proximal phalanx are predrilled with the provided 2.0-mm drill bit. Specific broaches are then used to expand the opening for the implant (**Fig. 2**). One broach is designed for use on the proximal phalanx and the other on the middle phalanx. Care should be taken to make sure the correct broach is used, as the design of these broaches is counterintuitive; the longer broach is for the middle phalanx whereas the shorter broach is for the proximal phalanx. The implant is grasped with forceps, and first inserted into the proximal phalanx and then the middle phalanx. The arthrodesis site is manually compressed for the next minute while the implant expands and engages cortical bone.[3]

The Smart Toe implant, like all the other newer implant devices, offers several advantages over traditional percutaneous K-wire fixation. Because the implant is internal and not protruding through the patient's digit, these implants have psychological advantages and reduce postoperative need for pin removal. Internal fixation eliminates pin tract infection, reduces the chance of inadvertent fixation removal, eliminates traumatic injury to the distal interphalangeal joint (DIPJ), and allows for a smaller postoperative dressing. The Smart Toe's one-piece compressive feature theoretically reduces the risk of nonunions while its shape prevents rotation of the implant.[3] Disadvantages include longer insertion time, increased costs, difficult removal, and the inconvenience of prior arrangements with the company representative.

To the authors' knowledge, only one article exists in the literature that assesses the Smart Toe implant. In 2009, Roukis[4] published a study in which 10 patients underwent 30 PIPJ fusions using Smart Toe fixation. All patients were neuropathic secondary to

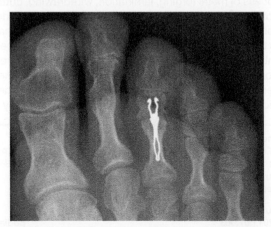

Fig. 1. Postoperative radiograph of Smart Toe. (*Courtesy of* John Ruch DPM, Tucker, GA.)

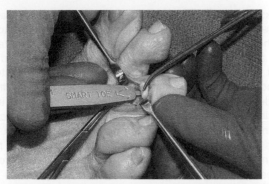

Fig. 2. Broaching technique during Smart Toe insertion. (*Courtesy of* John Ruch DPM, Tucker, GA.)

diabetes and underwent concurrent surgical procedures. Twenty-eight of the 30 digits went on to successful arthrodesis with a radiographic fusion rate of 93% at 10.2 months. The remaining patients who did not fuse went on to have a successful outcome and did not require implant removal.

HAMMERLOCK

The HammerLock (BioMedical Enterprises, Inc, San Antonio, TX, USA) digital implant is also a one-piece, NiTinol composite that uses metal memory technology (**Fig. 3**). The HammerLock implant comes in lengths of 16, 19, and 22 mm (corresponding to sizes small, medium, and large). The device is available in the straight design or with 10° plantarflexion. The proximal and distal segments are available in varying widths and lengths.[5] The distal segment width measures 6 mm (size small) or 6.5 mm (sizes medium and large). The proximal segment width measures 5.5 mm (size small) or 6.5 mm (size medium and large). The proximal segment length measures 5.5, 6.5, or 7.0 mm, which corresponds to small, medium, and large implants. The distal segment length measures 10, 12.5, or 15 mm, respectively.

The HammerLock insertion is similar to that of the Smart Toe. On PIPJ resection, the proximal and middle phalanx medullary canals are predrilled and broached. Custom forceps are used to remove the implant from its polyethylene storage housing, called

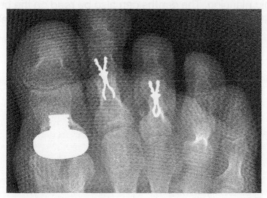

Fig. 3. Postoperative radiograph of HammerLock. (*Courtesy of* Thomas Brosky, DPM, Oakwood, GA.)

the HammerBlock; it is necessary that the implant is kept at less than 0°C for at least 30 minutes before removing the implant from the polyethylene storage block. The HammerLock is then inserted into the proximal phalanx. The clear tab on the implant is then removed and the distal portion of the implant is inserted into the middle phalanx. The joint is manually compressed for the next 1 to 2 minutes.[5]

The HammerLock has similar advantages and disadvantages to the other implantable PIPJ arthrodesis devices. The HammerBlock maintains the implant at cooler temperatures during the no-touch insertion of the device, allowing the surgeon up to 4 minutes for insertion. The clear tab component of the implant housing ensures that the implant is not inserted too far proximally into the proximal phalanx (**Fig. 4**).[5] Relative to the Smart Toe, the HammerLock has barbs on its proximal and distal components. These barbs are designed to maintain compression while minimizing stress on the cortical walls. Because the HammerLock has more barbs than the Smart Toe, it may theoretically engage more cortical bone when activated. This process may result in either increased implant stability or increased stress riser formation and cortical fracture. This feature may also make it more difficult to remove the implant if that situation were to arise. To the authors' knowledge, there is no published research on the HammerLock.

ARROW-LOK

The Arrow-Lok Digital Fusion System (Arrowhead Medical Device Technologies, Collierville, TN, USA) is another option for stable intramedullary fixation for PIPJ arthrodesis. The Arrow-Lok is a stainless-steel implant with a 3-dimensional barbed arrowhead design on its proximal and distal ends that function to engage compacted cancellous bone. Because this implant does not use metal memory technology, it does not require special handling or storage preoperatively or intraoperatively. The Arrow-Lok is available in lengths of 13, 16, 19, and 22 mm. The implant is also offered with a straight design or 10° plantarflexion. The apex is located slightly distal to accommodate for the shorter intramedullary canal in the middle phalanx. The central shaft diameter is 1.5 mm (0.059 in), providing strength to the device while not being so thick that it may cause stress risers (**Fig. 5**).[6]

The insertion of the Arrow-Lok is relatively straightforward and there are no time constraints on implant insertion. Following resection of the PIPJ, a reamer is used to create pilot holes in the intramedullary canals of both proximal and middle phalanges. Both phalanges are then broached to the depth estimated during preoperative radiographic planning. The depths can also be read on the broach; the depths corresponding to the proximal and middle phalanges are added together to determine

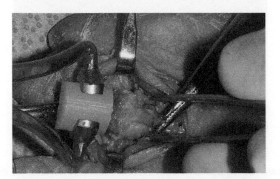

Fig. 4. HammerLock insertion demonstrating the function of the clear tab.

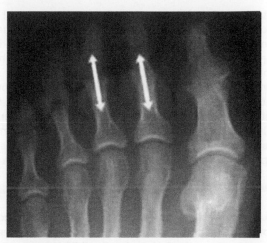

Fig. 5. Postoperative radiograph of Arrow-Lok. (*Courtesy of* Scott Roman, DPM, Covington, GA.)

the total length for the implant. The Arrow-Lok device is then implanted using insertion forceps and the digit is manually compressed to hold the arthrodesis in its final locked position. If removal is required at a later time, a similar surgical approach is used. Once the implant is exposed at the joint level, a wire-cutter is used to cut the shaft centrally. Then bone is resected around the implant with a side-cutting power burr or a 3.5-mm cannulated drill bit. The shaft is grasped with a straight hemostat or needle-nose pliers and removed from the intramedullary canal.[6]

To date no research has been published, due to the product's recent unveiling in February 2011. However, preliminary studies have shown that the Arrow-Lok has a pull-out strength of 22 N, almost 11 times that of a K-wire, when tested in bone models and polyurethane blocks. Also, the implant provides a rotational resistance of 19 N, more than 10 times that of a K-wire. In addition, 4-point bend testing, conducted by the Georgia Institute of Technology's Mechanical Properties Research Laboratory, revealed that K-wires were similar in fatigue failure. Overall, the Arrow-Lok appears to be a viable option for secure intramedullary fixation without time limitation on implant insertion; however, additional clinical studies are needed to demonstrate its efficacy.[6]

PRO-TOE VO HAMMERTOE FIXATION SYSTEM

The Pro-Toe VO Hammertoe Fixation System (Wright Medical Technology, Inc, Arlington, TN, USA) is a one-piece stainless-steel implant that provides secure, multiaxial fixation. The Pro-Toe VO has a threaded end proximally and a blade-style multibarbed end distally. This device has been designed to optimally engage intramedullary bone. Two lengths are available: 13 and 16 mm. The blade length and width are 6.5 and 4.0 mm, respectively. The 13-mm implant has a thread diameter of 2.0 mm and core diameter of 1.1 mm. The 16-mm implant has a thread diameter of 2.4 mm and core diameter of 1.6 mm. The implant is also offered with a straight design or with 10° plantarflexion.[7]

Once PIPJ joint surfaces are resected, the 0.045-in (1.1 mm) K-wire from the instrument kit is used to predrill both the proximal and middle phalanx intramedullary canals. Laser markings on the K-wire measure the depth of the proximal phalanx portion to determine the implant size. Only the middle phalanx is broached and fully seated until the shoulders contact the resection margin. Maintaining a uniplanal orientation while broaching allows optimal fit of the blade-style end. The appropriately sized implant is then engaged into the custom driver by aligning the laser marking on the blade with the angle markings on the driver head. The threaded end of the Pro-Toe VO is inserted into the proximal phalanx until it is fully seated. The laser markings should face dorsally prior to disengagement of the implant to ensure proper alignment. Once disengaged by squeezing a silicone O-ring on the driver head, the barbed blade end is inserted into the middle phalanx until the joint margins are flush. Multiple implants can be inserted with the same driver. Otherwise the instrumentation is single-use, eliminating facility cleaning and sterile processing.[7] As yet his product has no long-term published results, as it was recently introduced in March 2011.

STAYFUSE

The StayFuse (Nexa Orthopaedics, San Diego, CA, USA) is a two-piece titanium screw device designed for PIPJ fixation.[8] The two components snap together at the resected PIPJ to provide stability across the fusion site. The MID, or male, component corresponds with the middle phalanx and the PROX, or female, component corresponds with the proximal phalanx. The male component has a fluted section, which allows the device to flex enough to allow a straight ratcheting insertion of the male component into the female component. The two components have an interlocking thread pattern that secures them together (**Fig. 6**).

The design of the device and the use of minimal instrumentation aids in the ease of inserting the implant. The system provides a transparent template for radiograph overlay to determine implant size preoperatively. The surgeon must take into account the amount of shortening expected by joint resection.[8,9] The StayFuse system comes in various sizes that correspond to color schemes. Gold implants are designed for hallux interphalangeal joint fusion and have a 6.5-mm screw diameter. Gray implants are designed for lesser digits and come in screw diameters of 3.3, 3.8, 4.3, and 5.0 mm. Blue implants are available for smaller lesser digits and are available in screw diameters of 2.8, 3.8, and 4.3 mm.[8,9]

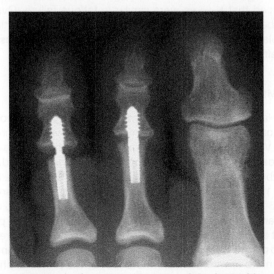

Fig. 6. Postoperative radiograph of StayFuse. (*Courtesy of* Charles Peebles, DPM, Atlanta, GA.)

After PIPJ resection, the proximal and middle phalanges' intramedullary canals are predrilled. The drill bit is advanced centrally into each canal until the shoulder stops the advancement. The two components are then inserted. First, the PROX component is inserted with the hex driver by hand or using a power drill. The PROX component is driven until it is flush with the distal aspect of the proximal phalanx. The MID component is then inserted, with care taken to assure it is aligned with the slot in the sagittal plane of the PROX component; this aligns the two components so they can snap together. The PIPJ is distracted to allow for separation of the two components to assure they are properly aligned. Moderate compression is then applied across the PIPJ and the implant is slightly rotated until the hexes engage. Forceful compression is then used to snap the components together so that the joint is properly aligned. The manufacturer recommends using intraoperative fluoroscopy to verify proper placement and length of the implant.[8]

The StayFuse device has advantages and disadvantages similar to other implantable PIPJ fixation devices. The StayFuse device is designed to provide rotational stability. However, determination of implant size prior to joint resection may lead to inaccurate implant sizing and subsequent pistoning of the implant in the bone.[8] If implant removal is necessary, a dorsal window is created over the middle phalanx and, using a small curette, the tip of the implant can be elevated and removed.[9,10] In 2010, Ellington and colleagues[10] performed a retrospective study on 38 toes over 31 months using the StayFuse device. The study reported that overall PIPJ alignment was maintained in 82% of patients, and none of the patients required a second procedure to remove the device. Although these investigators determined the StayFuse is efficacious for maintaining alignment, further evaluation is needed with longer follow-up periods postoperatively.

CANNULATED DIGITAL SCREWS

Cannulated screw fixation for digital arthrodesis is another PIPJ fixation option. Advantages of cannulated screw fixation are similar to the other implantable devices reviewed. Major disadvantages of cannulated screw fixation are screw breakage, distal tuft sensitivity, a toe that is too straight because of a rigid DIPJ, or a floating toe.

Cannulated screws can be inserted via DIPJ-sparing or DIPJ-stabilizing techniques.[11,12] The DIPJ-sparing technique involves inserting the cannulated screw from the DIPJ across the PIPJ fusion site. Countersinking the head of middle phalanx is necessary to avoid screw-head irritation. Mallet digit contracture is the main postoperative complication with this technique. Fibrosis at the DIPJ can be augmented by maintaining the guide wire in place for 2 to 4 weeks, and this can help to maintain the digit in its corrected position.[11]

The DIPJ-stabilizing technique requires screw entry from the distal aspect of the digit. The cannulated screw head is buried into the distal tuft of the distal phalanx, and the screw transverses the DIPJ and PIPJ fusion site. Mallet digit complications are avoided by using this technique because the DIPJ is sacrificed to fuse the PIPJ. The main disadvantage to this technique is the increased risk of the need for a second operation because of the persistent pain at the tip of the digit caused by the prominent screw head.[11,13]

Three companies offer cannulated digital fusion systems: OsteoMed (OsteoMed L.P., Addison, TX, USA), Ascension (Ascension Orthopedics, Austin, TX, USA), and Metasurg (Koby Ventures Ltd, Houston, TX, USA). Both Ascension and Metasurg offer 2.0 mm cannulated screws made of titanium alloy in lengths ranging from 24 to 50 mm. The OsteoMed system provides 2.0 mm cannulated screws measuring 20 to 42 mm in length and 2.4-mm cannulated screws measuring 28 to 50 mm in length. All of these screws have low-profile heads to prevent soft-tissue irritation.[14–16]

In 2004, Caterini and colleagues[13] conducted a retrospective review of 24 patients with 51 hammertoe deformities corrected by PIPJ arthrodesis with intramedullary titanium cannulated screw fixation using the DIPJ-stabilizing technique. The study reported a high success rate at an average of 2.6 years postoperatively. The investigation concluded there was a reduction in residual malalignment, decreased risk of mallet digit deformity, decreased risk of nonunion at the PIPJ, and fewer postoperative shoe restrictions relative to percutaneous K-wire fixation. Additional prospective study with longer follow-up and a larger sample size is necessary.

TRADITIONAL TECHNIQUES FOR DIGITAL FIXATION
Peg and Hole

In 1910, Soule described PIPJ arthrodesis as a surgical treatment for hammertoe deformity.[17] The procedure was first performed through a plantar incision. Without internal fixation, compression of the resected joint was achieved by maintaining the digit in dorsiflexion via cast immobilization for 6 weeks.[17] Sir Robert Jones introduced the dorsal incision approach in 1917.[18] The peg-in-hole arthrodesis technique, introduced by Higgs in 1931,[19] was described to be a more stable procedure that required non–weight bearing for only 3 weeks. Higgs fashioned the head of the proximal phalanx into a point and impacted it into the base of the middle phalanx to provide compression and stability. In 1938, Young[20] presented a modification of the peg-in-hole technique in which the proximal phalanx head was fashioned into a dowel rod, which was inserted into a hole in the middle phalanx base. Maintaining the dorsal cortex of the dowel rod intact provided increased strength to the fusion interface. Young claimed that the inherent stability of the fusion site negates the demand of internal fixation. The peg-in-hole design has been suggested to allow faster bone healing in comparison with end-to-end fusion because there is a larger cancellous bone interface.[21] Alvine and Garvin[22] reported a 97% fusion rate when using these techniques. However, difficulty of these procedures, shortening, the ease of fracture, and numerous other postoperative complications have led surgeons to increase the stability of the arthrodesis site via internal fixation.

Percutaneous K-Wire Fixation

Taylor[23] and Selig[24] recommended K-wire fixation to stabilize PIPJ arthrodesis in 1940 and 1941, respectively. This procedure allows the digit to function as a rigid lever on which the long flexor and extensor tendons can stabilize the metatarsophalangeal joint (MPJ).[25] Secure internal fixation allows for relatively earlier mobilization and ambulation.[24]

Postoperatively, motion across the PIPJ must be eliminated until bone union is achieved. This action is necessary because K-wire fixation allows pistoning, does not prevent frontal plane rotation, and does not provide compression. Fusion is typically seen after 6 to 8 weeks of using a postoperative surgical shoe. The stiff-soled surgical shoe eliminates the propulsive phase of gait, and this maintains position and prevents motion that could cause stress on the K-wire.[26] A noncompliant patient who does not use the postoperative surgical shoe could fatigue or fracture K-wires.[27,28] In addition, the sight of a surgical shoe and the pins protruding from the distal digit may remind the patient and nearby people of the recent surgery and the need to maintain a decreased activity level despite a reduction of painful symptoms. Pins extruding out the digit can be problematic if they become caught on the patient's bandage, bed sheets, and so forth. Inadvertent immature removal of the K-wires is a concern that should be prevented. The digits may be completely covered with dressings to prevent this; however, this makes initial postoperative vascular assessment of the digits difficult. Another potential but rare complication of using percutaneous K-wire fixation is pin tract infection, and this too requires visualization of the digit for diagnosis.

The long-term assessment by Coughlin and colleagues[29] of 118 PIPJ arthrodeses (63 patients) at an average of 61 months of follow-up concluded that PIPJ arthrodesis with K-wire fixation is a reliable procedure that consistently yields satisfactory results. Bone fusion was achieved in 81% of digits and fibrous union in the remaining 19%. Pain relief was accomplished in 92% of patients, and patient satisfaction was 84%. Lemm and colleagues[30] reported a similar rate of patient satisfaction, at 86%. Malalignment (15%) and numbness (6%) have been associated with unsuccessful results.[29] Poor dissection technique, excessive motion postoperatively, or failure to maintain the bone surfaces in contact may explain these complications. Dorsal contracture can result from excessive scarring and fibrosis; however, this can be minimized by bandaging the digit in slight plantarflexion and by providing patients with postoperative range-of-motion exercises.[28]

Buried K-Wire Fixation

In 1995, Creighton and Blustein[31] introduced the buried K-wire technique for PIPJ arthrodesis. This technique can prevent the postoperative complications of traditional K-wire fixation, such as pin tract infection. Creighton and Blustein inserted the K-wire as previously described for the traditional K-wire insertion approach; however, they made a stab incision at the distal aspect of the digit, bent the K-wire, and pressed the K-wire against the tuft of the distal phalanx as it was retrograded proximally.

In 2008, Camasta and Cass[32] presented a modified buried K-wire technique. This technique is different in that the K-wire is first inserted from the PIPJ to the base of the proximal phalanx, cut 5 to 10 mm distal to the proximal phalanx, and then seated into a predrilled hole in the base of the middle phalanx (**Figs. 7** and **8**). Before cutting the wire, a plantarflexory bend can be applied to the wire to allow the arthrodesis to appear more natural. The technique then involves skewering the exposed K-wire into position on the middle phalanx. This technique offers several advantages relative to the previously reported techniques. Like the newer and more expensive fixation approaches, this cost-conscious method eliminates skin compromise of the digit distally, eliminates pin tract infection, reduces early inadvertent K-wire removal, reduces bending or fracture of the K-wire, and does not require unnecessarily induced arthritis of the DIPJ.[32] Camasta's group retrospectively reviewed 50 PIPJ arthrodeses (37 patients) using his buried K-wire technique and reported 100% clinical fusion and 96% radiographic union by postoperative week 9. Two delayed unions (4%) and one proximal pin migration (2%) were reported; however, no patient required fixation removal or revisional surgery (Camasta CA, Cass AD, Dalmia L. Arthrodesis of the proximal interphalangeal joint using buried kirschner wires. Submitted for publication). These findings suggest this fixation technique is comparable, if not superior, to other fixation methods. Overall, the buried K-wire technique is safe, simple, effective, and cost-conscious[32] (Camasta CA, Cass AD, Dalmia L. Arthrodesis of the proximal interphalangeal joint using buried kirschner wires. Submitted for publication).

With regard to which K-wire to use, several options are available. Different K-wire diameters may be used depending on the size of the digit and whether the metatarsophalangeal joint is also being fixated. A 0.045-in (1.14 mm) smooth K-wire is used commonly for PIPJ arthrodesis. If this diameter is loose in the bone, a 0.054-in (1.4 mm) or 0.062-in (1.6 mm) K-wire can be used. Adequate size is necessary to provide

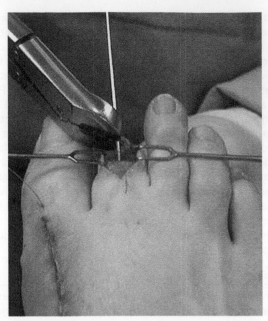

Fig. 7. Buried K-wire technique. The K-wire is inserted into the proximal phalanx, bent, cut 5 to 10 mm past the arthrodesis site, skewered onto the middle phalanx, and compressed. (*Courtesy of* Craig Camasta, DPM, Atlanta, GA.)

joint stability, but care should be taken to avoid using excessively large-diameter wires that could cause vascular compromise. The diameter of K-wire will affect the ease of bending and cutting it during the procedure. Although stainless-steel K-wires are commonly used, titanium K-wires are available for use in patients with a nickel allergy. Absorbable fixation options are also available for patients with nickel allergy.

Absorbable Fixation

Absorbable intramedullary pins have several reported advantages over traditional percutaneous K-wire fixation. The absorbable pins are somewhat flexible, and this allows them to be bent into predrilled holes in the head of the proximal phalanx and base of the middle phalanx. As described for the buried K-wire technique, burying absorbable fixation has several advantages. Konkle and colleagues[33] performed PIPJ arthrodesis with 2.0-mm Orthosorb (Resorbable Pin poly-P-Dioxanone and D&C Violet #2 distributed by DePuy, Ace Medical, Warsaw, IN, USA) fixation on 48 digits over a mean follow-up of 39 months, and reported 8% unsuccessful results. Floating digits were associated with Weil osteotomies on the same toes, and transverse plane deviations were attributed to using pins that were too small in diameter. However, it was reported that larger-diameter pins are not available. Burns and Varin[34] reported 6 cases of digital arthrodesis fixated with Biofix (polyglycolic acid distributed by Kirschner Medical Corp, since acquired by Biomet Inc, Warsaw, IN, USA) fixation with no reported infection, fixation failure, osteolytic change, or development of sinus tract. These good outcomes are supported by Pietrzak and colleagues,[35] who demonstrated that biodegradable hammertoe implants have similar biomechanical properties to stainless-steel K-wires throughout a 6-week postoperative course. Arthrex Inc (Naples, FL, USA) continues to produce bioabsorbable K-wires in 1.5- and 2.0-mm diameters; the 1.5-mm diameter is slightly smaller than a 0.062-in (1.57 mm) K-wire

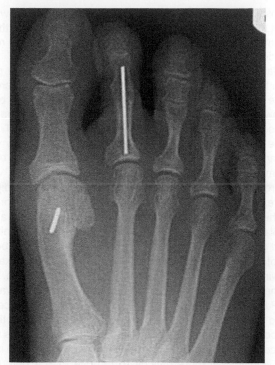

Fig. 8. Radiograph of a second PIPJ arthrodesis with buried K-wire fixation. (*Courtesy of* Craig Camasta, DPM, Atlanta, GA.)

and can be used for digital fusion fixation when indicated. Although absorbable fixation may offer several advantages, general disadvantages include decreased strength over time, increased cost, and potential for undesired biological response.[36] Augmentation of absorbable pins by suturing a Vicryl loop through predrilled holes in the proximal phalanx head and middle phalanx base has been suggested.[37,38] A similar technique has been outlined for PIPJ fixation using stainless-steel monofilament suture in an intraosseous loop fashion, with or without K-wire fixation.[26,38] This technique is reported to be easy to perform and resistant to displacement; however, clinical data have not yet been presented.[38]

DISCUSSION

Significant advancements have recently been made in digital surgery. Newer fixation devices appear to be establishing themselves as useful options. With the recent appearance of these products, foot and ankle surgeons are forced to reanalyze more traditional types of fixation and compare those with these new devices. When critically evaluating any implant device, it is important to consider surgical technique, cost, potential complications, patient expectations, and surgical outcomes.

Digital surgery is a technical exercise, and requires dexterity and attention to detail. Obtaining adequate exposure of the PIPJ, while not compromising the neurovascular status of the digit, is critical and arguably more important than the method of arthrod esis fixation. Once the joint is exposed, proper resection is then necessary. Hand instrumentation can be used to resect the joint while maintaining length and a contoured apposition of the two bone surfaces. Saw resection allows good bone-to-bone contact, but may compromise length. Careful preservation of the collateral ligaments during joint dissection allows for later collateral ligament reapproximation, which affords added stability to the arthrodesis.

Digital arthroplasty has a role for hammertoe correction. These procedures may initially straighten the digit, but effectively destabilize the digit and create an environment for possible deformity recurrence. DIPJ arthroplasties may be an adjunctive procedure for claw digit deformities in conjunction with PIPJ arthrodesis.

The cost of these newer devices is a topic of significant concern. Traditional fixation of the hammertoe deformity with K-wires has been used for many years with good surgical results, and K-wires are inarguably inexpensive. The cost of using a K-wire is roughly $7 compared with the cost of a newer implant device, which is roughly $1000. This difference in cost is magnified when fixating multiple digits of the same patient. Therefore, reimbursement will be a determining factor for the surgeon in choosing his or her preferred type of fixation. If a surgeon seeks a cost-conscious and effective implantable device that combines advantages and minimizes disadvantages of new and old fixation methods, buried K-wire fixation may be optimal.

Conversely, potential disadvantages of percutaneous K-wire fixation include pin tract infection, wire breakage, bending, and lack of compression.[10] Psychological disturbance to the patient, the need for postoperative wire removal, and traumatic injury to the DIPJ can be eliminated by using implantable devices. Using digital implants may lead to better outcomes and increased patient satisfaction through elimination of these potential complications.[10] Although newer implants seem to provide a better fixation, complications may still arise. When implant removal is required, these devices may be significantly more difficult to remove than a percutaneous K-wire. Some companies have specific removal techniques for their implant, although the level of difficulty surrounding removal remains unknown. **Fig. 9** demonstrates a Smart Toe that was inserted through the PIPJ and unintentionally entered the DIPJ. The distal arms of the implant are longer than the middle phalanx. Techniques that require determination of implant length preoperatively may predispose these problems to occur; preoperative radiographic assessment may be helpful, but implant length is ideally determined intraoperatively after joint resection. If the proximal phalanx is not drilled or broached far enough proximally, the implant will be positioned more distal and the distal component will extend farther than intended. Because excessive overdrilling

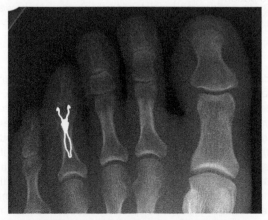

Fig. 9. Radiograph demonstrating complication using Smart Toe.

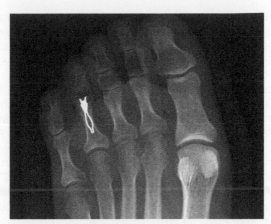

Fig. 10. Postoperative radiograph after revision of Smart Toe complication.

or broaching may allow an implant to piston and violate the MPJ or DIPJ, implant preparation must be precise. Regardless of the reason, this patient developed pain at the DIPJ, which needed to be readdressed surgically. **Fig. 10** shows the postoperative radiograph after a DIPJ arthroplasty was performed with an oscillating saw. The surgeon cut the distal barbs, rather than interrupting the arthrodesis site and removing the entire implant. The patient no longer has pain at the DIPJ and is satisfied with the surgical outcome.

SUMMARY

Many fixation options are currently available for digital PIPJ arthrodesis. The newer intramedullary implants are becoming an accepted method of fixation for this procedure. These implants may seem functional in theory; however, long-term research is required before any strong conclusions for their success may be drawn. Until this research is available, surgeons' anecdotal experience and familiarity with fixation techniques may guide their preferred fixation method. Both percutaneous K-wire fixation and the newer implants have advantages and disadvantages. Therefore, many variables must be considered when deciding on what fixation device should be used for a specific patient. Cost, patient compliance, and patient expectations should be considered. K-wires remain the current standard for the PIPJ arthrodesis, and should be a readily available technique for all surgeons in the case of an implant failure.

REFERENCES

1. Glissan DJ. The indications for inducing fusion at the ankle joint by operation with description of two successful techniques. Aust N Z J Surg 1949;19:64–71.
2. Memometal Incorporation USA. Smart Toe intramedullary shape memory implant [brochure]. 2009. Available at: www.mmi-usa.com. Accessed March 21, 2011.
3. Memometal Incorporation USA. Foot and ankle: Smart Toe—shape memory intramedullary implant. 2010. Available at: http://uk.memometal.com/products/foot_ankle/smart-toe.html. Accessed March 21, 2011.
4. Boukis TS. A 1-piece shape-metal nitinol intramedullary internal fixation device for arthrodesis of the proximal interphalangeal joint in neuropathic patients with diabetes. Foot Ankle Spec 2009;2(3):130–4.

5. BioMedical Enterprises, Inc. HammerLock nitinol intramedullary fixation system [brochure]. 2010. Available at: www.bme-tx.com. Accessed March 21, 2011.

6. Arrowhead Medical Device Technologies, LLC. Arrow-Lok digital fusion system [brochure]. 2011. Available at: www.arrowheaddevices.com. Accessed March 21, 2011.

7. Wright Medical Technology, Inc. Pro-Toe VO hammertoe implant system [brochure]. 2011. Available at: www.wmt.com. Accessed March 21, 2011.

8. Nexa Orthopedics, Tornier Dx. StayFuse intramedullary fusion device [brochure]. 2011. Available at: www.tornierdx.com/stayfuse/interdigital.php. Accessed March 21, 2011.

9. Yu GV, Vincent AL, Khoury WE, et al. Techniques of digital arthrodesis: revisiting the old and discovering the new. Clin Podiatr Med Surg 2004;21:17–50.

10. Ellington JK, Anderson RB, Davis WH, et al. Radiographic analysis of proximal interphalangeal joint arthrodesis with an intramedullary fusion device for lesser toe deformities. Foot Ankle Int 2010;31(5):372–6.

11. Good J, Fiala K. Digital surgery: current trends and techniques. Clin Podiatr Med Surg 2010;27:583–99.

12. Lane GD. Lesser digital fusion with a cannulated screw. J Foot Ankle Surg 2005; 44(3):249.

13. Caterini R, Farsetti P, Tarantino U, et al. Arthrodesis of the toe joints with an intramedullary cannulated screw for correction of hammertoe deformity. Foot Ankle Int 2004;25(4):256–61.

14. Ascension Orthopedics. Capture screw system—digital fusion screws. 2011. Available at: www.ascensionortho.com. Accessed March 21, 2011.

15. OsteoMed. Cannulated screws for digital arthrodesis. 2011. Available at: www.osteomedcorp.com. Accessed March 21, 2011.

16. MetaSurg. Titanium digital fusion system. 2011. Available at: www.metasurg.com. Accessed March 21, 2011.

17. Soule RE. Operation for the cure of hammertoe. N Y Med J 1910;91:649.

18. Jones R. Notes on military orthopaedics. New York: P.B. Hoeber; 1917. p. 38.

19. Higgs SL. Hammer-toe, 131. Medical Press; 1931. p. 473.

20. Young CS. An operation for the correction of hammer-toe and claw-toe. J Bone Joint Surg 1938;20:715.

21. Schelfman BS, Fenton CF, McGlamry ED. Peg in hole arthrodesis. J Am Podiatry Assoc 1983;73:187–95.

22. Alvine FG, Garvin KL. Peg and dowel fusion of the proximal interphalangeal joint. Foot Ankle 1980;1(2):190–4.

23. Taylor RG. An operative procedure for the treatment of hammer-toe and claw-toe. J Bone Joint Surg 1940;22:608.

24. Selig S. Hammer-toe: a new procedure for its correction. Surg Gynecol Obstet 1941;72:101.

25. Banks AS, Downey MS, Martin DE, et al, editors. McGlamry's comprehensive textbook of foot and ankle surgery. 3rd edition. Philadelphia: Lippincott Williams & Wilkins; 2001.

26. Gerbert J. Digital arthrodesis. Clin Podiatry 1985;2(1):81–94.

27. Fenton CF. Postoperative management following digital surgery. J Am Podiatr Med Assoc 1985;75(1):36–41.

28. Monson DK, Buell TR, Scurran BL. Lesser digital arthrodesis. Clin Podiatr Med Surg 1986;3(2):347–56.

29. Coughlin MJ, Dorris J, Polk E. Operative repair of the fixed hammertoe deformity. Foot Ankle Int 2000;21(2):94–104.

30. Lemm M, Green R, Green D. Summary of retrospective long-term review of proximal interphalangeal joint arthroplasty and arthrodesis procedures for hammertoe correction. In: Ruch JA, editor. Reconstructive surgery of the foot and leg. Update '96. Tucker (GA): Podiatry Institute; 1996. p. 194–6.
31. Creighton RE, Blustein SM. Buried Kirschner wire fixation in digital fusion. J Foot Ankle Surg 1995;34:567–70.
32. Camasta CA, Cass AD. Buried Kirschner-wire fixation for hammertoe arthrodesis. In: Miller SJ, editor. Reconstructive surgery of the foot and leg. Update 2008. Tucker (GA): Podiatry Institute; 2008. p. 5–8.
33. Konkel KF, Menger AG, Retzlaff SA. Hammer toe correction using an absorbable intramedullary pin. Foot Ankle Int 2007;28(8):916–20.
34. Burns AE, Varin J. Poly-L-lactic acid rod fixation results in foot surgery. J Foot Ankle Surg 1998;37(1):37–41.
35. Pietrzak WS, Lessek TP, Perns SV. A bioabsorbable fixation implant for use in proximal interphalangeal joint (hammer toe) arthrodesis: biomechanical testing in a synthetic bone substrate. J Foot Ankle Surg 2006;45(5):288–94.
36. Ambrose CG, Clanton TO. Bioabsorbable implants: review of clinical experience in orthopedic surgery. Ann Biomed Eng 2004;32(1):171–7.
37. Giovinco JD. End-to-end arthrodesis with absorbable pin and suture fixation. Clin Podiatr Med Surg 1996;13:251–4.
38. Harris W IV, Mote GA, Malay DS. Fixation of the proximal interphalangeal arthrodesis with the use of an intraosseous loop of stainless-steel wire suture. J Foot Ankle Surg 2009;48(3):411–4.

Index

Note: Page numbers of article titles are in **boldface** type.

A

Absorbable fixation, for hammertoe, 778–779
Achilles tendon
  involved in midfoot collapse, 680
  lengthening of, with subtalar arthroereisis, 750
  rupture of, percutaneous fixation of, 722–723
Agility ankle implant, 739–740
Allgöwer, Martin, 608
Allgower dynamic compression plates, 622
Ankle
  fractures of, percutaneous fixation of, 720
  total replacement of. *See* Total ankle replacement.
Ankle evolutive system, 738
AO (Arbeitsgemeinschaft für Osteosynthesefragen), founding of, 608
AO calcaneal plate, 700
Arbeitsgemeinschaft für Osteosynthesefragen, founding of, 608
Arrow-Lok implant, 772–773
Arthritis
  total ankle replacement for, 728–732
  total first metatarsophalangeal joint arthroplasty for, **755–761**
Arthrodesis
  digital, **769–783**
  first metatarsal cuneiform, anatomic-specific plates for, 692
  first metatarsal phalangeal, anatomic-specific plates for, 690–691
  Lisfranc, anatomic-specific plates for, 693–695
  tibiotalocalcaneal, intramedullary nail fixation for, **633–648**
Arthroereisis, subtalar, **745–754**
Arthroplasty, first metatarsophalangeal joint, **755–761**
Aseptic loosening, in total ankle replacement, 738
Association for the Study of Internal Fixation (ASIF), founding of, 608
Axial screw fixation, for Charcot arthropathy, 678
Axis altering arthroereisis implants, 747

B

Bagby, George, 612
Bioabsorbable arthroereisis implants, 747
Bircher, H., 611
Böhler, Lorenz, 610
Bone, healing of, 713
Bone grafts, in intramedullary nail fixation, 635–636

Clin Podiatr Med Surg 28 (2011) 785–794
doi:10.1016/S0891-8422(11)00090-5
0891-8422/11/$ – see front matter © 2011 Elsevier Inc. All rights reserved.

P

R

United States Postal Service

Statement of Ownership, Management, and Circulation
(All Periodicals Publications Except Requestor Publications)

1. Publication Title	2. Publication Number	3. Filing Date
Clinics in Podiatric Medicine & Surgery	0 0 0 - 7 0 7	9/16/11

4. Issue Frequency	5. Number of Issues Published Annually	6. Annual Subscription Price
Jan, Apr, Jul, Oct	4	$270.00

7. Complete Mailing Address of Known Office of Publication (Not printer) (Street, city, county, state, and ZIP+4®)

Elsevier Inc.
360 Park Avenue South
New York, NY 10010-1710

Contact Person
Stephen Bushing

Telephone (Include area code)
215-239-3688

8. Complete Mailing Address of Headquarters or General Business Office of Publisher (Not printer)

Elsevier Inc., 360 Park Avenue South, New York, NY 10010-1710

9. Full Names and Complete Mailing Addresses of Publisher, Editor, and Managing Editor (Do not leave blank)

Publisher (Name and complete mailing address)

Kim Murphy, Elsevier, Inc., 1600 John F. Kennedy Blvd. Suite 1800, Philadelphia, PA 19103-2899

Editor (Name and complete mailing address)

Patrick Manley, Elsevier, Inc., 1600 John F. Kennedy Blvd. Suite 1800, Philadelphia, PA 19103-2899

Managing Editor (Name and complete mailing address)

Barton Dudlick, Elsevier, Inc., 1600 John F. Kennedy Blvd. Suite 1800, Philadelphia, PA 19103-2899

10. Owner (Do not leave blank. If the publication is owned by a corporation, give the name and address of the corporation immediately followed by the names and addresses of all stockholders owning or holding 1 percent or more of the total amount of stock. If not owned by a corporation, give the names and addresses of the individual owners. If owned by a partnership or other unincorporated firm, give its name and address as well as those of each individual owner. If the publication is published by a nonprofit organization, give its name and address.)

Full Name	Complete Mailing Address
Wholly owned subsidiary of	4520 East-West Highway
Reed/Elsevier, US holdings	Bethesda, MD 20814

11. Known Bondholders, Mortgagees, and Other Security Holders Owning or Holding 1 Percent or More of Total Amount of Bonds, Mortgages, or Other Securities. If none, check box ☐ None

Full Name	Complete Mailing Address
N/A	

12. Tax Status (For completion by nonprofit organizations authorized to mail at nonprofit rates) (Check one)
The purpose, function, and nonprofit status of this organization and the exempt status for federal income tax purposes:
☐ Has Not Changed During Preceding 12 Months
☐ Has Changed During Preceding 12 Months (Publisher must submit explanation of change with this statement)

PS Form 3526, September 2007 (Page 1 of 3 Instructions Page 3)) PSN 7530-01-000-9931 PRIVACY NOTICE: See our Privacy policy in www.usps.com

---

13. Publication Title	14. Issue Date for Circulation Data Below
Clinics in Podiatric Medicine & Surgery	July 2011

15. Extent and Nature of Circulation		Average No. Copies Each Issue During Preceding 12 Months	No. Copies of Single Issue Published Nearest to Filing Date
a. Total Number of Copies (Net press run)		1184	1148
b. Paid Circulation (By Mail and Outside the Mail)	(1) Mailed Outside-County Paid Subscriptions Stated on PS Form 3541. (Include paid distribution above nominal rate, advertiser's proof copies, and exchange copies)	660	595
	(2) Mailed In-County Paid Subscriptions Stated on PS Form 3541 (Include paid distribution above nominal rate, advertiser's proof copies, and exchange copies)		
	(3) Paid Distribution Outside the Mails Including Sales Through Dealers and Carriers, Street Vendors, Counter Sales, and Other Paid Distribution Outside USPS®	49	51
	(4) Paid Distribution by Other Classes Mailed Through the USPS (e.g. First-Class Mail®)		
c. Total Paid Distribution (Sum of 15b (1), (2), (3), and (4))		709	646
d. Free or Nominal Rate Distribution (By Mail and Outside the Mail)	(1) Free or Nominal Rate Outside-County Copies Included on PS Form 3541	75	76
	(2) Free or Nominal Rate In-County Copies Included on PS Form 3541		
	(3) Free or Nominal Rate Copies Mailed at Other Classes Through the USPS (e.g. First-Class Mail)		
	(4) Free or Nominal Rate Distribution Outside the Mail (Carriers or other means)		
e. Total Free or Nominal Rate Distribution (Sum of 15d (1), (2), (3) and (4))		75	76
f. Total Distribution (Sum of 15c and 15e)		784	722
g. Copies not Distributed (See instructions to publishers #4 (page #3))		400	426
h. Total (Sum of 15f and g)		1184	1148
i. Percent Paid (15c divided by 15f times 100)		90.43%	89.47%

16. Publication of Statement of Ownership

☐ If the publication is a general publication, publication of this statement is required. Will be printed in the October 2011 issue of this publication. ☐ Publication not required

17. Signature and Title of Editor, Publisher, Business Manager, or Owner

Stephen R. Bushing   Date September 16, 2011

Stephen R. Bushing – Inventory/Distribution Coordinator

I certify that all information furnished on this form is true and complete. I understand that anyone who furnishes false or misleading information on this form or who omits material or information requested on the form may be subject to criminal sanctions (including fines and imprisonment) and/or civil sanctions (including civil penalties).

PS Form 3526, September 2007 (Page 2 of 3)

Moving?

Make sure your subscription moves with you!

To notify us of your new address, find your **Clinics Account Number** (located on your mailing label above your name), and contact customer service at:

Email: journalscustomerservice-usa@elsevier.com

800-654-2452 (subscribers in the U.S. & Canada)
314-447-8871 (subscribers outside of the U.S. & Canada)

Fax number: 314-447-8029

Elsevier Health Sciences Division
Subscription Customer Service
3251 Riverport Lane
Maryland Heights, MO 63043

*To ensure uninterrupted delivery of your subscription, please notify us at least 4 weeks in advance of move.

Printed and bound by CPI Group (UK) Ltd, Croydon, CR0 4YY

03/10/2024

01040458-0001